Disclaimer: The information presented in this book is intended for general educational and informational purposes only. It is not intended to be a substitute for professional medical advice, diagnosis, or treatment. Always seek the advice of your physician or other qualified healthcare provider with any questions you may have regarding a medical condition. The author and publisher of this book are not responsible for any adverse effects or consequences resulting from the use of the information in this book. The information presented in this book is based on the author's personal experiences and research, and should not be considered as medical advice or a substitute for professional medical care. The author and publisher do not make any warranties or representations regarding the completeness, accuracy, or reliability of the information presented in this book. The reader assumes all risks and responsibilities for any decisions or actions taken based on the information presented in this book.

Chapter 1: Introduction to Losing Weight

Losing weight is a journey that requires dedication, commitment, and effort. It's a journey that can be challenging, but it's also one of the most rewarding things you can do for your health and well-being. Whether you're looking to lose a few pounds or a significant amount of weight, it's important to understand that there is no quick fix or magic solution. Losing weight requires a lifestyle change that includes healthy eating habits, regular exercise, and a positive mindset.

The first step in losing weight is to understand why it's important. Excess weight can lead to a variety of health problems, including heart disease, diabetes, high blood pressure, and joint pain. Losing weight can also boost your energy levels, improve your mood, and increase your self-confidence. It's not just about fitting into your favorite jeans or looking good in a swimsuit – it's about improving your overall quality of life.

Before you begin your weight loss journey, it's important to assess your current habits and lifestyle. This includes taking an honest look at your diet, physical activity level, and overall health. It's also important to set realistic goals and expectations. Losing weight is not a one-size-fits-all process, and everyone's journey will be different. It's important to focus on progress, not perfection, and celebrate small victories along the way.

One of the keys to successful weight loss is to make sustainable changes to your lifestyle. This means finding healthy eating habits and exercises that work for you, and that you enjoy. It's important to remember that weight loss is not about depriving yourself of your favorite foods or punishing yourself with strenuous exercise. It's about finding a balance that works for you and your body.

Throughout this book, we'll explore the various aspects of losing weight, including healthy eating habits, exercise, mindset, and more. We'll provide practical tips and strategies for incorporating healthy habits into your lifestyle and staying motivated throughout your journey.

Whether you're just getting started or you've been on the weight loss journey for a while, this book will provide valuable insights and guidance to help you reach your goals.

Chapter 2: Understanding Your Body Mass Index (BMI)

When it comes to losing weight, understanding your body mass index (BMI) is an important first step. BMI is a measure of body fat based on your weight in relation to your height. It's a useful tool for determining whether you're at a healthy weight, overweight, or obese.

To calculate your BMI, you can use a BMI calculator or the following formula:

BMI = weight (kg) / height^2 (m^2)

If you're using pounds and inches, you can use the following formula:

BMI = (weight in pounds / height in inches^2) x 703

Once you have calculated your BMI, you can use the following guidelines to determine where you fall on the BMI scale:

A BMI of less than 18.5 is considered underweight

A BMI between 18.5 and 24.9 is considered normal weight

A BMI between 25 and 29.9 is considered overweight

A BMI of 30 or higher is considered obese

While BMI is a useful tool for estimating body fat, it's important to note that it has limitations. For example, it doesn't take into account factors such as muscle mass or body composition. Someone with a lot of muscle mass, for example, may have a higher BMI but still be considered healthy.

In addition to BMI, it's also important to measure your waist circumference. Carrying excess weight around your waist is associated with an increased risk of health problems such as heart disease and type 2 diabetes.

To measure your waist circumference, use a measuring tape to measure around your waist at your belly button. For women, a waist circumference of more than 35 inches (88 cm) is considered high risk. For men, a waist circumference of more than 40 inches (102 cm) is considered high risk.

By understanding your BMI and waist circumference, you can get a better sense of where you stand in terms of your weight and health. If you fall into the overweight or obese categories, losing weight can have a significant impact on your health and wellbeing. By setting realistic weight loss goals and adopting healthy habits, you can work towards achieving a healthy weight and reducing your risk of weight-related health problems.

Chapter 3: Setting Realistic Weight Loss Goals

Setting goals is an essential part of any weight loss journey. Without a clear plan and objectives, it can be difficult to stay motivated and track progress. However, it's important to set realistic weight loss goals to ensure success and avoid disappointment or frustration.

When setting weight loss goals, it's important to consider your starting point, your overall health, and your lifestyle. Rapid weight loss may seem appealing, but it can be unhealthy and unsustainable in the long term. Aiming for a slow and steady weight loss of 1-2 pounds per week is a healthy and realistic goal for most people.

It's also important to set specific and measurable goals. Rather than just saying you want to lose weight, set a target weight or a specific amount of weight to lose over a certain time frame. This will help you track your progress and stay motivated as you see yourself getting closer to your goal.

Another important consideration when setting weight loss goals is your overall health and wellbeing. Focusing solely on weight loss can lead to unhealthy habits and behaviors, such as crash dieting or over-exercising. Instead, focus on developing healthy habits, such as eating a balanced diet and incorporating regular physical activity into your daily routine. These habits will not only support weight loss but also improve your overall health and wellbeing.

It's also important to be flexible with your weight loss goals. Life can be unpredictable, and there may be times when your weight loss progress stalls or you face challenges that make it difficult to stick to your plan. Don't be too hard on yourself if this happens – it's normal to experience setbacks along the way. Instead, reevaluate your goals and adjust them as needed to ensure they remain realistic and achievable.

In summary, setting realistic weight loss goals is essential for success on your weight loss journey. Consider your starting point, overall health, and lifestyle when setting goals, and aim for a slow and steady weight loss of 1-2 pounds per week. Set specific and measurable goals, and focus on developing healthy habits rather than just losing weight. Finally, be flexible with your goals and adjust them as needed to ensure they remain realistic and achievable.

Chapter 4: Benefits of Losing Weight

Losing weight can have a multitude of benefits beyond simply looking better in your clothes. In fact, the benefits of weight loss extend far beyond cosmetic reasons and can have a significant impact on your overall health and well-being. Here are just a few of the many benefits of losing weight:

Improved Heart Health: Losing weight can significantly reduce your risk of heart disease, stroke, and other cardiovascular diseases. By shedding excess pounds, you can lower your blood pressure, reduce your cholesterol levels, and decrease your risk of developing heart disease.

Increased Energy Levels: Carrying extra weight can make everyday activities more challenging and leave you feeling tired and sluggish. By losing weight, you can improve your overall energy levels and feel more motivated to stay active and engage in physical activity.

Improved Sleep Quality: Losing weight can improve the quality and duration of your sleep. Sleep apnea, a condition where breathing is briefly interrupted during sleep, is often associated with obesity. By losing weight, you can reduce your risk of developing sleep apnea and improve your sleep quality overall.

Reduced Joint Pain: Excess weight can put additional strain on your joints, particularly in the knees and hips. By losing weight, you can reduce the pressure on your joints and alleviate joint pain and stiffness.

Improved Mental Health: Losing weight can also have a positive impact on your mental health. People who are overweight or obese are at a higher risk for depression and other mental health issues. By losing weight, you can improve your self-esteem and confidence, which can lead to improved mental health and well-being.

Reduced Risk of Chronic Diseases: Obesity is a risk factor for a variety of chronic diseases, including type 2 diabetes, certain types of cancer, and liver disease. By losing weight, you can reduce your risk of developing these conditions and improve your overall health.

Improved Quality of Life: Losing weight can lead to an overall improvement in your quality of life. You may find that you have more energy, feel more confident in your appearance, and are able to engage in activities that you were previously unable to do.

Overall, the benefits of losing weight go far beyond cosmetic reasons. By shedding excess pounds, you can improve your overall health and well-being, reduce your risk of chronic diseases, and improve your quality of life.

Chapter 5: Choosing the Right Weight Loss Plan for You

When it comes to losing weight, there is no one-size-fits-all solution. Choosing the right weight loss plan for you can be overwhelming, but it's important to find a plan that fits your lifestyle, preferences, and goals. In this chapter, we'll explore some of the most popular weight loss plans and provide tips on how to choose the right one for you.

Consider Your Goals: The first step in choosing the right weight loss plan is to determine your weight loss goals. Do you want to lose weight quickly or gradually? Do you have a specific target weight in mind? Knowing your goals can help you determine which weight loss plan is best for you.

Assess Your Lifestyle: Your lifestyle plays a major role in choosing a weight loss plan. Are you a busy person who needs quick and easy meal options? Do you have time for meal preparation and cooking? Consider your lifestyle when choosing a plan that will fit into your routine.

Evaluate Your Eating Habits: Do you have any dietary restrictions or preferences? Some weight loss plans require you to eliminate certain food groups, while others allow for more flexibility. Consider your eating habits and preferences when choosing a plan that you can stick to long-term.

Research Different Plans: There are countless weight loss plans available, each with its own approach and philosophy. Do your research and learn about the different plans, including their success rates, potential risks, and benefits. Some popular plans include:

Low-carb diets: These diets focus on reducing carbohydrates and increasing protein and fat intake.

Mediterranean diets: These diets emphasize whole, unprocessed foods such as fruits, vegetables, whole grains, and lean protein.

Intermittent fasting: This approach involves alternating periods of fasting and eating.

Meal replacement plans: These plans involve replacing one or more meals per day with shakes, bars, or other pre-packaged meals.

Weight loss programs: These programs provide guidance, support, and accountability, and may include meal plans, exercise plans, and counseling.

Consult with a Professional: If you have any underlying health conditions or concerns, it's important to consult with a healthcare professional before starting a weight loss plan. They can help you determine which plan is safe and effective for you, and provide guidance on how to adjust your plan to meet your needs.

Remember, the most effective weight loss plan is one that you can stick to long-term. Choosing a plan that fits your lifestyle, preferences, and goals will increase your chances of success and help you achieve your desired results.

Chapter 6: The Role of Exercise in Weight Loss

When it comes to losing weight, diet and exercise go hand in hand. While a healthy diet is essential for weight loss, incorporating exercise into your routine can help you burn more calories, build muscle, and boost your metabolism. In this chapter, we'll discuss the role of exercise in weight loss and provide tips for incorporating physical activity into your weight loss plan.

Why Exercise Is Important for Weight Loss

Exercise plays a crucial role in weight loss for several reasons. First, it burns calories. When you exercise, your body uses energy to power your muscles. The more intense the exercise, the more calories you'll burn. This energy deficit can help you lose weight over time.

Second, exercise can help you build muscle. Muscle is more metabolically active than fat, which means that it burns more calories at rest. By building more muscle through exercise, you can boost your metabolism and burn more calories throughout the day.

Finally, exercise can help you maintain your weight loss over time. Regular physical activity has been shown to improve weight maintenance and reduce the risk of weight regain.

What Types of Exercise Are Best for Weight Loss?

When it comes to exercise for weight loss, there's no one-size-fits-all approach. The best type of exercise for you depends on your preferences, fitness level, and weight loss goals. However, here are some types of exercise that can be particularly effective for weight loss:

Cardiovascular exercise: This type of exercise gets your heart rate up and burns calories. Examples include running, cycling, swimming, and dancing.

High-intensity interval training (HIIT): This type of exercise involves short bursts of intense exercise followed by periods of rest. HIIT workouts can help you burn a lot of calories in a short amount of time.

Strength training: This type of exercise involves using weights or resistance to build muscle. As we mentioned earlier, building muscle can boost your metabolism and help you burn more calories at rest.

Low-intensity steady-state (LISS) cardio: This type of exercise involves doing a low-intensity activity, such as walking or biking, for an extended period of time. While it may not burn as many calories as high-intensity exercise, it can still be an effective way to increase your daily activity level and burn calories.

Tips for Incorporating Exercise into Your Weight Loss Plan

If you're new to exercise, it's important to start slowly and gradually increase your activity level. Here are some tips for incorporating exercise into your weight loss plan:

Start small: If you're not used to exercising, start with just a few minutes of activity each day and gradually work your way up.

Find activities you enjoy: Exercise doesn't have to be a chore. Find activities that you enjoy, whether it's hiking, swimming, or dancing.

Make it a habit: Set a schedule for your workouts and stick to it. Consistency is key when it comes to seeing results from exercise.

Mix it up: Don't do the same workout every day. Mix up your routine with different types of exercise to challenge your body and prevent boredom.

Get support: Enlist the help of a friend or family member to exercise with you. Having a workout buddy can provide motivation and accountability.

Conclusion

Exercise is an important part of any weight loss plan. By incorporating physical activity into your routine, you can burn more calories, build muscle, and boost your metabolism. Remember to start slowly, find activities you enjoy, and make exercise a habit. With time and consistency, you'll start to see the benefits of exercise for weight loss.

Chapter 7: Healthy Eating Habits for Weight Loss

When it comes to losing weight, what you eat is just as important as how much you eat. Developing healthy eating habits is essential for sustainable weight loss and overall health. Here are some healthy eating habits you can incorporate into your daily routine:

Eat a balanced diet: A balanced diet includes a variety of fruits, vegetables, whole grains, lean proteins, and healthy fats. Eating a variety of nutrient-dense foods ensures that your body gets the vitamins and minerals it needs to function properly.

Control portion sizes: Portion control is key when it comes to weight loss. Use smaller plates and bowls, and measure your food to ensure you're not overeating.

Eat mindfully: Pay attention to your body's hunger and fullness cues. Eat slowly and savor each bite. Avoid distractions like watching TV or using your phone while eating.

Stay hydrated: Drinking plenty of water helps you feel full and can prevent overeating. Aim for at least 8 glasses of water a day.

Plan and prepare meals: Planning and preparing meals in advance can help you make healthier choices and avoid impulse eating. Set aside time each week to plan your meals and grocery shop.

Limit processed foods: Processed foods are often high in calories, sugar, and unhealthy fats. Try to limit your intake of processed foods and opt for whole, unprocessed foods whenever possible.

Snack wisely: Snacking can be a healthy part of your diet, but it's important to choose nutritious snacks like fruits, vegetables, and nuts. Avoid snacks that are high in sugar, salt, or unhealthy fats.

Be mindful of sugar and salt intake: Too much sugar and salt can contribute to weight gain and other health problems. Be mindful of the sugar and salt content in your food and opt for lower-sugar and lower-sodium options whenever possible.

Remember, developing healthy eating habits takes time and effort. Start by making small changes to your diet and gradually incorporate more healthy habits into your routine. Making sustainable changes to your eating habits will not only help you lose weight but will also improve your overall health and well-being.

Chapter 8: Mindful Eating Techniques

One of the most important things you can do when trying to lose weight is to pay attention to what you eat and how you eat it. Mindful eating techniques can help you do just that. By being more present and focused during meals, you can enjoy your food more, feel more satisfied, and avoid overeating.

Here are some mindful eating techniques to try:

Slow Down: It's easy to rush through meals without really tasting or enjoying the food. Instead, try to eat slowly and savor each bite. Put your fork down between bites, and take a deep breath or two. This will help you be more mindful of your food, and also give your brain time to register that you're full.

Pay Attention to Your Senses: Take time to notice the smells, tastes, textures, and colors of your food. This can help you appreciate and enjoy it more, and also tune in to your body's hunger and fullness signals.

Avoid Distractions: Eating while watching TV, reading, or working can make it harder to pay attention to your food and how much you're eating. Instead, try to eat in a quiet, calm environment where you can focus on your meal.

Listen to Your Body: Check in with your body throughout the meal to see how hungry or full you feel. Stop eating when you're comfortably full, even if there's still food on your plate. It can also be helpful to wait a few minutes before deciding if you want seconds, to see if you're still hungry or if you're satisfied.

Practice Gratitude: Take a moment to express gratitude for your food and the people who helped bring it to you. This can help you feel more positive and present during meals, and also foster a sense of connection and gratitude.

Engage Your Senses: Engage all of your senses in the eating experience. Take note of the sound of the food as you bite into it, the way it feels in your mouth, and the way it smells. This will help you be more mindful of what you are eating, and may help you appreciate it more.

By practicing these mindful eating techniques, you can help break the cycle of mindless eating and develop a more positive relationship with food. This can not only help you lose weight but also improve your overall quality of life.

Chapter 9: The Importance of Hydration in Weight Loss

Water is essential for life and it is also an essential part of any successful weight loss plan. Hydration plays a critical role in many of our body's functions, including metabolism, digestion, and nutrient absorption. In fact, staying hydrated can be one of the most important factors when it comes to losing weight and maintaining a healthy body weight.

When our bodies are dehydrated, it can lead to a number of negative consequences. For example, dehydration can cause our metabolism to slow down, which means our body burns fewer calories. Additionally, dehydration can cause our bodies to hold onto excess water weight, which can make us feel bloated and uncomfortable.

One of the most important benefits of staying hydrated is that it can help to curb our appetite. Many times when we feel hungry, we may actually just be thirsty. Drinking water before meals can help us to feel full more quickly, which can help us to eat less overall.

Another benefit of staying hydrated is that it can help to increase our energy levels. When we are dehydrated, we often feel tired and lethargic. This can make it difficult to stick to our weight loss plan, as we may not have the energy to exercise or prepare healthy meals.

So, how much water should we be drinking? The answer varies depending on our age, weight, and activity level. However, a good general guideline is to aim for at least eight 8-ounce glasses of water per day. Additionally, we should try to drink water throughout the day, rather than trying to drink it all at once.

If you find it difficult to drink enough water, there are a few things you can try. First, try adding flavor to your water by infusing it with fresh fruit or herbs. You can also try drinking sparkling water or seltzer if you prefer carbonation. Finally, try carrying a water bottle with you throughout the day, so that you can sip on water whenever you feel thirsty.

In summary, staying hydrated is a critical part of any weight loss plan. It can help to increase our energy levels, curb our appetite, and promote healthy metabolism and digestion. So, don't forget to drink up and stay hydrated!

Chapter 10: Meal Planning and Preparation Tips

One of the most effective ways to lose weight is by planning and preparing your meals ahead of time. Meal planning and preparation can help you save time, reduce stress, and make healthy eating a habit. Here are some meal planning and preparation tips to help you stay on track with your weight loss goals:

Set aside time for meal planning: Dedicate some time each week to plan your meals for the upcoming week. This will help you save time and money, and reduce the stress of figuring out what to eat each day.

Choose healthy and balanced meals: When planning your meals, make sure to choose a variety of healthy and balanced foods that include lean protein, whole grains, fruits, and vegetables. This will help you stay full and satisfied, while providing your body with the nutrients it needs.

Use a meal planner: Use a meal planner to map out your meals for the week. This can be as simple as a notebook or as high-tech as a meal planning app.

Make a grocery list: After you've planned your meals for the week, make a grocery list of all the ingredients you'll need. Stick to your list when you go grocery shopping to avoid buying unhealthy or unnecessary items.

Batch cook: Prepare large batches of healthy meals at once and freeze them for later. This will save you time and ensure that you always have healthy meals on hand.

Prep ingredients in advance: Prepare ingredients in advance, such as washing and chopping vegetables or cooking grains and proteins, to save time during the week.

Use portion control: Use portion control when preparing and serving your meals. This can help you avoid overeating and stick to your weight loss goals.

Experiment with new recipes: Try new recipes to keep your meals interesting and enjoyable. Look for healthy recipes online or in cookbooks.

Pack your own meals: When eating out or at work, pack your own healthy meals and snacks. This will help you avoid unhealthy options and stay on track with your weight loss goals.

Stay flexible: Remember that meal planning and preparation is a tool to help you reach your weight loss goals, but it's okay to be flexible and make adjustments when needed. Listen to your body and make changes that work for you.

By taking the time to plan and prepare your meals, you can make healthy eating a habit and achieve your weight loss goals. Experiment with different meal planning and preparation techniques to find what works best for you.

Chapter 11: Tracking Your Progress and Staying Accountable

Tracking your progress and staying accountable is an important aspect of losing weight. It helps you to stay motivated, identify areas of improvement, and measure your success. In this chapter, we'll explore why tracking your progress is important, how to track your progress effectively, and how to stay accountable to yourself and others.

Why Tracking Your Progress is Important

Tracking your progress can help you in a number of ways. First and foremost, it allows you to see how far you've come. It's easy to lose sight of your progress when you're in the thick of it, but by tracking your progress, you can see how much weight you've lost, how many inches you've lost, or how much your fitness level has improved.

This can be a powerful motivator and help you stay focused on your weight loss goals.

Tracking your progress can also help you identify areas of improvement. For example, if you're tracking your food intake and notice that you're consistently going over your calorie goal, you can adjust your diet accordingly. Similarly, if you're tracking your exercise routine and notice that you're not seeing the results you want, you can switch up your workout routine.

How to Track Your Progress

There are many different ways to track your progress. Some common methods include:

Keeping a food diary: This involves writing down everything you eat and drink throughout the day, along with the calorie count.

Measuring your body: This involves measuring your weight, body fat percentage, and/or inches lost.

Using a fitness tracker: This involves using a device or app to track your physical activity, such as steps taken, calories burned, and heart rate.

Taking progress photos: This involves taking photos of yourself at regular intervals to see how your body is changing over time.

It's important to choose a tracking method that works for you and that you can stick to. Some people prefer to use an app or device, while others find that writing things down on paper works best for them. Whatever method you choose, make sure it's something that you can easily incorporate into your daily routine.

Staying Accountable

Staying accountable to yourself and others is an important part of the weight loss journey. Here are a few strategies for staying accountable:

Set goals: Set specific, measurable goals for yourself and track your progress towards those goals.

Find a workout buddy: Having a workout partner can help keep you motivated and accountable. You can push each other to work harder and celebrate your successes together.

Join a support group: Joining a weight loss support group can provide you with a sense of community and accountability. You can share your successes and struggles with others who are going through the same thing.

Hire a coach: Working with a coach or personal trainer can provide you with expert guidance and accountability. They can help you stay on track and make adjustments to your plan as needed.

Conclusion

Tracking your progress and staying accountable are essential components of a successful weight loss journey. By tracking your progress, you can see how far you've come and identify areas of improvement. And by staying accountable, you can stay motivated and committed to your weight loss goals. Use the strategies outlined in this chapter to track your progress and stay accountable to yourself and others.

Chapter 12: Understanding Portion Sizes

When it comes to losing weight, one of the most important things you can do is understand portion sizes. This is because eating too much of any type of food, even healthy foods, can lead to weight gain. But how do you know how much you should be eating? Here are some tips to help you understand portion sizes and make healthier choices.

Use visual cues

One of the easiest ways to understand portion sizes is to use visual cues. For example, a serving of protein, such as meat, chicken or fish, should be about the size of a deck of cards or the palm of your hand. A serving of grains, such as rice or pasta, should be about the size of your fist. And a serving of fruits or vegetables should be about the size of a tennis ball.

Read labels

Another way to understand portion sizes is to read food labels. Many packaged foods, such as cereals, snacks, and drinks, have information on the label about serving sizes. Pay attention to the serving size, as well as the number of servings per container, and make sure you're not eating more than the recommended amount.

Use measuring cups and spoons

Using measuring cups and spoons is another way to help you understand portion sizes. This is especially helpful when cooking or preparing food at home. For example, measuring out one serving of rice or pasta can help you avoid overeating.

Practice mindful eating

Practicing mindful eating can also help you understand portion sizes. This means paying attention to your hunger and fullness cues, and eating slowly and without distractions. When you're more in tune with your body, you're less likely to overeat.

Be mindful of restaurant portions

Finally, when eating out at restaurants, be mindful of portion sizes. Many restaurants serve large portions that can be two or three times the recommended serving size.

Consider sharing a meal with a friend or taking half of the meal home for leftovers.

Understanding portion sizes is key to making healthier choices and losing weight. By using visual cues, reading labels, using measuring cups and spoons, practicing mindful eating, and being mindful of restaurant portions, you can make sure you're eating the right amount of food for your body.

Chapter 13: Strategies for Eating Out and Social Gatherings

Social gatherings and eating out can be some of the biggest challenges to sticking with your weight loss plan. The temptation to indulge in unhealthy foods and drinks can be overwhelming, and it can be difficult to make healthy choices when surrounded by so many tempting options. However, with a little planning and preparation, you can successfully navigate these situations and stay on track with your weight loss goals.

Do Your Research

Before going out to eat, research the restaurant's menu and nutrition information online. Look for healthier options that fit within your dietary guidelines and caloric limits. Many restaurants now offer lighter or healthier menu options, so take advantage of those choices.

Plan Ahead

If you know you'll be going out to eat or to a social gathering, plan ahead by eating a small, healthy snack beforehand. This can help curb your appetite and prevent overeating.

Focus on Protein and Vegetables

When you're at the restaurant or social gathering, make sure to fill up on protein and vegetables first. Choose dishes that are high in lean protein, such as grilled chicken or fish, and opt for vegetables as your side dish.

Be Mindful of Portions

Portion sizes at restaurants can be much larger than what you would normally eat at home. Be mindful of how much you're consuming and consider splitting a meal with a friend or taking leftovers home.

Avoid Liquid Calories

Alcoholic and sugary beverages can quickly add up in calories and hinder your weight loss progress. Opt for water, unsweetened tea or coffee, or a light beverage instead.

Don't Deprive Yourself

It's important to enjoy yourself and indulge in moderation. If there's a specific dish or treat that you've been looking forward to, allow yourself to have it in a small portion.

Practice Mindful Eating

Take your time and savor your food. Put your fork down between bites and chew slowly. This will help you to better recognize when you're full and avoid overeating.

Avoid Eating Late at Night

Eating late at night can sabotage your weight loss efforts. Try to eat at least two to three hours before bedtime, and if you do need a snack, choose something small and healthy like a piece of fruit or a handful of nuts.

By implementing these strategies, you can successfully navigate eating out and social gatherings while still staying on track with your weight loss goals. Remember to enjoy yourself, but also be mindful of your choices and portions.

Chapter 14: Healthy Snack Ideas

Snacking is an important part of our daily routine, but it can also be a challenge when trying to lose weight. Many of us reach for snacks that are high in calories, sugar, and unhealthy fats, which can derail our weight loss efforts. But snacking doesn't have to be a diet disaster! Here are some healthy snack ideas that are both satisfying and weight loss friendly:

Apple slices with almond butter: This snack is a great combination of healthy carbs, fiber, and protein. The apple provides natural sweetness, while the almond butter adds healthy fats and protein.

Hummus and vegetable sticks: Hummus is a great source of protein and healthy fats, and pairing it with crunchy vegetable sticks like carrots, celery, or bell peppers makes for a satisfying and low-calorie snack.

Greek yogurt with berries: Greek yogurt is a great source of protein, and adding fresh or frozen berries provides natural sweetness and antioxidants.

Rice cakes with avocado: Rice cakes are a low-calorie and crunchy snack, and pairing them with mashed avocado adds healthy fats and fiber.

Hard boiled eggs: Eggs are a great source of protein and nutrients, and hard boiled eggs make for a convenient and portable snack.

Roasted chickpeas: Chickpeas are a great source of plant-based protein and fiber, and roasting them with spices like cumin, paprika, or chili powder makes for a crunchy and satisfying snack.

Air-popped popcorn: Popcorn is a low-calorie and high-fiber snack, and air-popping it instead of using microwave popcorn with added fats and salt makes it even healthier.

Cottage cheese with sliced peaches: Cottage cheese is a great source of protein, and adding sliced peaches provides natural sweetness and fiber.

Trail mix: Make your own trail mix by combining nuts, seeds, and dried fruits for a satisfying and nutrient-dense snack.

Edamame: Edamame is a great source of plant-based protein and fiber, and steaming or boiling them with a sprinkle of salt makes for a simple and healthy snack.

Remember, snacks can be a part of a healthy and sustainable weight loss plan. The key is to choose snacks that are nutrient-dense and satisfy your hunger, while avoiding snacks that are high in calories, sugar, and unhealthy fats. With these healthy snack ideas, you can snack smart and support your weight loss goals.

Chapter 15: Identifying and Avoiding Emotional Eating Triggers

Food can be a source of comfort and pleasure for many people, and it's common to turn to food in times of stress, sadness, or other emotional states. Emotional eating, however, can lead to overeating and weight gain. In this chapter, we will discuss how to identify emotional eating triggers and strategies for avoiding them.

Identifying Emotional Eating Triggers

The first step in avoiding emotional eating is to identify your personal triggers. Ask yourself these questions to help identify when you may be at risk for emotional eating:

Do I tend to eat more when I'm feeling stressed, anxious, or sad?

Do I eat when I'm bored or lonely?

Do certain people, situations, or emotions trigger my desire to eat?

Do I tend to crave specific foods when I'm emotional?

Am I more likely to eat when I'm watching TV or using my phone?

Once you've identified your personal triggers, you can start working on strategies to avoid them.

Avoiding Emotional Eating Triggers

Here are some strategies to help you avoid emotional eating triggers:

Keep a Food Journal: Keeping a food journal can help you identify patterns in your eating habits and emotions. This can help you recognize when you're eating for emotional reasons and give you a chance to change your behavior.

Practice Mindful Eating: Mindful eating involves paying attention to your food and your body's hunger and fullness cues. By being present and aware during meals, you can avoid using food as a distraction or coping mechanism.

Find Alternative Coping Mechanisms: Rather than turning to food when you're feeling emotional, find other ways to cope. Exercise, meditation, deep breathing, or talking to a friend or therapist can all be effective alternatives.

Remove Trigger Foods: If you know certain foods are a trigger for emotional eating, remove them from your home or workplace. If you're out and about and craving a trigger food, try to distract yourself with a healthier option or a non-food activity.

Create a Support System: Surrounding yourself with supportive friends and family members can help you avoid emotional eating. They can offer encouragement and accountability, and may be able to help you identify triggers you hadn't recognized before.

By identifying your emotional eating triggers and implementing strategies to avoid them, you can take control of your eating habits and improve your overall health and well-being. Remember that change takes time and effort, but with practice, you can develop healthy habits that will serve you well for years to come.

Chapter 16: Incorporating More Vegetables and Fruits into Your Diet

Eating a diet rich in fruits and vegetables can help you achieve your weight loss goals while also providing essential nutrients and promoting overall health. Fruits and vegetables are low in calories but high in fiber, vitamins, and minerals, making them an ideal addition to any weight loss plan. In this chapter, we'll explore some easy ways to incorporate more fruits and vegetables into your diet.

Experiment with different types of fruits and vegetables: Many people get stuck in a rut of eating the same fruits and vegetables over and over again. Try branching out and experimenting with different types of produce. You might discover a new favorite that you never would have tried otherwise.

Add vegetables to your meals: Look for ways to add vegetables to your meals. For example, add spinach or kale to your morning smoothie, top your pizza with veggies like mushrooms and bell peppers, or mix shredded carrots or zucchini into your meatloaf or pasta sauce.

Snack on fruits and vegetables: Instead of reaching for processed snacks like chips or cookies, snack on fruits and vegetables. Keep cut-up veggies like carrots, cucumbers, and cherry tomatoes in the fridge for easy snacking, or grab an apple or banana on the go.

Swap out less healthy ingredients: Many recipes can be modified to include more fruits and vegetables. For example, swap out the pasta in your spaghetti dish for spaghetti squash or zucchini noodles, or replace half the meat in your chili with extra beans and veggies.

Try new cooking techniques: If you're not a fan of raw veggies, try cooking them in a new way. Roasting, grilling, and stir-frying can all bring out the natural sweetness and flavors in vegetables.

Make smoothies and juices: Smoothies and juices are a great way to pack in a lot of fruits and vegetables in one go. Experiment with different combinations to find a recipe that you love.

Incorporating more fruits and vegetables into your diet can be a simple and delicious way to support your weight loss goals. Whether you're adding them to your meals, snacking on them throughout the day, or experimenting with new recipes and cooking techniques, there are plenty of ways to make fruits and vegetables a staple in your diet.

Chapter 17: The Role of Protein in Weight Loss

When it comes to losing weight, many people focus on

reducing their caloric intake and increasing their physical activity. However, the role of protein in weight loss is often overlooked. Protein is a crucial nutrient that plays a vital role in weight loss and overall health. In this chapter, we'll explore the benefits of protein for weight loss and how to incorporate it into your diet.

Protein is an essential nutrient that helps to build and repair tissues, including muscles. It is also important for the production of enzymes, hormones, and other essential molecules in the body. When it comes to weight loss, protein is particularly beneficial because it helps to increase feelings of fullness and reduce cravings, which can lead to consuming fewer calories overall.

Studies have shown that a high-protein diet can lead to increased weight loss and reduced body fat compared to diets that are lower in protein. This is because protein has a higher thermic effect than carbohydrates or fats, which means that your body burns more calories digesting protein than it does digesting other nutrients. Additionally, protein helps to preserve lean muscle mass, which is important for maintaining a healthy metabolism and burning calories even when you're not exercising.

So, how much protein do you need to consume to reap the benefits for weight loss? The recommended daily intake of protein varies based on factors such as age, gender, and activity level. However, a general rule of thumb is to aim for at least 0.8 grams of protein per kilogram of body weight per day. For example, if you weigh 150 pounds, you would need to consume around 55 grams of protein per day.

To incorporate more protein into your diet, focus on consuming lean protein sources such as chicken, fish, turkey, tofu, legumes, and low-fat dairy products. These foods are not only high in protein but also tend to be lower in calories and saturated fat compared to other protein sources such as red meat. You can also add protein powder to smoothies or oatmeal for an extra boost of protein.

In summary, protein plays a critical role in weight loss and should not be overlooked when developing a weight loss plan. Aim to consume at least 0.8 grams of protein per kilogram of body weight per day and focus on lean protein sources such as chicken, fish, and tofu. By incorporating protein into your diet, you can help to increase feelings of fullness, reduce cravings, and preserve lean muscle mass, leading to increased weight loss and improved overall health.

Chapter 18: Strategies for Dealing with Food Cravings

Food cravings can be a major obstacle in any weight loss journey. When you have a strong craving for a certain food, it can be hard to resist, and this can sabotage your efforts to lose weight. However, there are strategies you can use to deal with food cravings and stay on track with your weight loss goals.

Identify the Triggers of Your Cravings

The first step in dealing with food cravings is to identify what triggers them. For some people, it may be stress, boredom, or even a certain time of day. Once you know what triggers your cravings, you can work on developing strategies to prevent them from occurring.

Keep Healthy Snacks on Hand

One way to deal with food cravings is to have healthy snacks on hand that you can turn to instead of indulging in unhealthy options. Stock your pantry and fridge with fresh fruits and vegetables, nuts, and other healthy snacks. This can help you satisfy your hunger without derailing your weight loss progress.

Practice Mindful Eating

Another strategy for dealing with food cravings is to practice mindful eating. This means paying attention to your food, enjoying it slowly, and savoring every bite. When you eat mindfully, you are more likely to feel satisfied and less likely to experience strong cravings for unhealthy foods.

Distract Yourself

When a food craving strikes, it can be helpful to distract yourself with a different activity. This can be as simple as going for a walk, doing some yoga, or calling a friend. By focusing on something else, you can take your mind off of your craving and avoid giving in to temptation.

Drink Water

Drinking water can also be an effective way to deal with food cravings. Sometimes, we mistake thirst for hunger, and simply drinking a glass of water can help us feel full and satisfied. Additionally, staying hydrated can help keep your cravings in check.

Plan for Occasional Treats

It's important to remember that indulging in a treat every once in a while is not going to ruin your weight loss progress. In fact, allowing yourself the occasional indulgence can help prevent feelings of deprivation and keep you motivated to stick to your healthy habits.

Seek Support

Finally, seeking support from friends, family, or a support group can be a helpful strategy for dealing with food cravings. By having someone to talk to and share your struggles with, you can stay accountable and motivated to reach your weight loss goals.

In conclusion, dealing with food cravings is an important aspect of any weight loss journey. By identifying your triggers, keeping healthy snacks on hand, practicing mindful eating, distracting yourself, drinking water, planning for occasional treats, and seeking support, you can overcome your cravings and stay on track with your weight loss goals.

Chapter 19: Overcoming Plateaus and Sticking with Your Plan

Have you ever experienced a weight loss plateau? It can be incredibly frustrating when you're putting in effort but the scale won't budge. The truth is, plateaus are a normal part of the weight loss journey. However, there are strategies you can use to overcome plateaus and stay motivated to achieve your goals.

The first step in overcoming a plateau is to reassess your plan. Are you still following the same routine as when you started your weight loss journey? Our bodies are incredibly adaptive, so it's possible that your body has adjusted to your current routine and is no longer responding to it. Consider changing up your exercise routine, increasing the intensity or duration of your workouts, or trying a new type of exercise altogether. Similarly, reassess your diet and consider tweaking your calorie intake, trying new healthy recipes, or experimenting with intermittent fasting.

Another important factor in overcoming a plateau is to stay motivated. Remember why you started your weight loss journey and visualize your goals. Celebrate the progress you have made so far, even if the scale isn't moving at the moment. Consider setting non-scale goals, such as increasing your strength or endurance, fitting into a certain piece of clothing, or improving your overall health.

It's also important to stay accountable. Track your food intake and exercise, and make sure you're staying within your daily calorie goals. Consider joining a weight loss support group or working with a personal trainer or nutritionist to stay on track and receive expert guidance.

Finally, remember to be patient with yourself. Weight loss is not always linear, and it may take time to break through a plateau. Keep in mind that your weight is just one aspect of your overall health, and focus on making sustainable lifestyle changes that will benefit your physical and mental health in the long run.

By reassessing your plan, staying motivated and accountable, and being patient with yourself, you can overcome plateaus and continue on your weight loss journey with renewed energy and focus.

Chapter 20: Building a Support System for Weight Loss

Losing weight can be a challenging journey, and it's important to have a support system in place to help you stay motivated and on track. Whether it's family, friends, or a professional, building a support system can make a big difference in your weight loss success.

Identify your Support System

The first step in building a support system is to identify the people in your life who can support your weight loss journey. This might include family members, close friends, co-workers, or even an online support group. Consider the people in your life who are positive, supportive, and have a genuine interest in your health and well-being.

Communicate Your Goals

Once you've identified your support system, it's important to communicate your weight loss goals and how they can help you achieve them. Be honest and open about what you're trying to achieve and how they can support you along the way. Let them know what kind of help you need, whether it's someone to exercise with, someone to talk to when you're feeling discouraged, or someone to share healthy meals with.

Find Accountability

Accountability is a key component of any successful weight loss journey. Consider finding a partner or group to help keep you accountable for your actions and progress. This could be a personal trainer, a weight loss coach, or even a friend who is also trying to lose weight. Having someone to report to and share progress with can be a powerful motivator.

Get Active Together

Exercise is an important part of any weight loss plan, and doing it with someone else can be even more motivating. Consider finding a workout buddy or joining a fitness class with a friend. Not only will this help you stay accountable and motivated, but it can also make exercise more enjoyable and fun.

Share Meals

Eating healthy meals is essential for weight loss, but it can also be challenging to do alone. Consider sharing meals with your support system, whether it's cooking together or sharing healthy recipe ideas. Having someone to share meals with can make healthy eating more enjoyable and help you stay on track.

Celebrate Successes

Finally, it's important to celebrate your successes along the way. Share your progress with your support system and celebrate milestones together. Whether it's a healthy meal out or a fun activity, finding ways to celebrate your successes can help keep you motivated and on track.

In summary, building a support system is an important part of any weight loss journey. Identify the people in your life who can support you, communicate your goals, find accountability, get active together, share meals, and celebrate successes. With a strong support system in place, you'll be well on your way to achieving your weight loss goals.

Chapter 21: The Benefits of Strength Training for Weight Loss

When it comes to losing weight, many people focus on cardio exercises and dieting alone. However, incorporating strength training into your weight loss plan can have numerous benefits. Here are just a few:

Increased Muscle Mass: Strength training helps to build and maintain lean muscle mass, which can help to increase your metabolism. This means that even when you're not working out, your body will be burning more calories than it would if you had less muscle mass.

Improved Body Composition: While losing weight can help you to lose fat, it can also lead to a loss of muscle mass if you're not careful. Strength training can help you to maintain your muscle mass while losing fat, which can lead to a more desirable body composition overall.

Reduced Risk of Injury: Strengthening your muscles can help to improve your balance and stability, reducing your risk of falls and other injuries. This can be especially important as you get older and become more susceptible to injury.

Increased Bone Density: Strength training has been shown to increase bone density, which can help to prevent osteoporosis and other bone-related conditions.

Improved Mental Health: Exercise in general has been shown to have numerous mental health benefits, and strength training is no exception. It can help to reduce stress, anxiety, and symptoms of depression, leading to an overall improvement in mood and mental wellbeing.

So if you're looking to lose weight, don't overlook the benefits of strength training. Even just a few sessions a week can make a significant difference in your weight loss journey. Be sure to talk to a trainer or other professional to develop a strength training plan that is safe and effective for you.

Chapter 22: Incorporating Cardiovascular Exercise into Your Routine

Cardiovascular exercise is one of the most effective ways to burn calories, increase your heart rate, and improve your overall health. Incorporating regular cardio exercise into your weight loss routine can help you achieve your weight loss goals more quickly and efficiently. In this chapter, we will discuss the benefits of cardiovascular exercise, how to get started with cardio, and how to incorporate cardio into your daily routine.

The Benefits of Cardiovascular Exercise

Cardiovascular exercise, also known as cardio, is any activity that increases your heart rate and breathing rate, such as running, cycling, swimming, or dancing. There are many benefits of cardiovascular exercise, including:

Burning calories: Cardio is one of the most effective ways to burn calories, which is essential for weight loss.

Strengthening your heart and lungs: Regular cardio can improve your heart and lung function, reducing your risk of heart disease, stroke, and other health problems.

Reducing stress and anxiety: Cardio is an excellent stress reliever and can improve your mood and mental health.

Improving sleep: Regular cardio can help you fall asleep faster and sleep more soundly.

Boosting energy levels: Cardio can increase your energy levels and reduce fatigue.

Getting Started with Cardio

If you're new to cardio exercise, it's essential to start slowly and gradually increase the intensity and duration of your workouts over time. It's also important to choose an activity that you enjoy, as you're more likely to stick with it if you enjoy it.

Some good options for beginners include:

Walking: Walking is a great way to get started with cardio exercise. It's low-impact, easy to do, and can be done almost anywhere.

Cycling: Cycling is a fun and low-impact way to get your heart rate up. You can cycle outdoors or on a stationary bike.

Swimming: Swimming is a great low-impact option that works your entire body.

As you become more comfortable with cardio exercise, you can gradually increase the intensity and duration of your workouts. Aim for at least 30 minutes of moderate-intensity cardio exercise most days of the week.

Incorporating Cardio into Your Daily Routine

One of the best ways to make sure you're getting enough cardio exercise is to incorporate it into your daily routine. Here are some tips for doing so:

Walk or bike to work: If possible, walk or bike to work instead of driving or taking public transportation.

Take the stairs: Instead of taking the elevator, take the stairs whenever possible.

Break up your day with short bursts of activity: Take a brisk walk during your lunch break or do some jumping jacks during commercial breaks while watching TV.

Schedule regular workouts: Make cardio exercise a priority by scheduling regular workouts into your calendar. Try to stick to a consistent schedule to make it a habit.

Conclusion

Incorporating regular cardiovascular exercise into your weight loss routine can help you achieve your goals more quickly and improve your overall health. Whether you prefer walking, cycling, swimming, or dancing, find an activity that you enjoy and make it a regular part of your routine. Remember to start slowly and gradually increase the intensity and duration of your workouts over time.

Chapter 23: Combining Exercise and Healthy Eating for Maximum Results

Losing weight is not just about cutting calories or exercising more. It's about finding a balance between healthy eating and physical activity that works for your body and your lifestyle. While diet and exercise are often seen as separate factors in weight loss, they are actually interrelated and can be combined for maximum results.

Exercise and healthy eating work together to help you achieve your weight loss goals. Exercise burns calories and boosts your metabolism, which can help you lose weight faster. Healthy eating, on the other hand, provides your body with the nutrients it needs to perform at its best during exercise.

When you combine exercise and healthy eating, you create a powerful synergy that can help you achieve your weight loss goals more quickly and efficiently. Here are some tips for combining exercise and healthy eating for maximum results:

Fuel up before exercise: Eating a healthy meal or snack before exercise can help you perform better and burn more calories. Aim to eat a combination of carbohydrates and protein before exercising to provide your body with the energy it needs.

Eat a balanced diet: Eating a balanced diet that includes plenty of fruits, vegetables, whole grains, lean protein, and healthy fats will provide your body with the nutrients it needs to perform at its best during exercise. It will also help you maintain a healthy weight over the long term.

Hydrate: Drinking enough water is essential for both exercise and weight loss. Aim to drink at least eight glasses of water a day, and more if you're exercising or sweating heavily.

Make exercise a regular part of your routine: Consistency is key when it comes to exercise. Make it a regular part of your routine, and aim to get at least 150 minutes of moderate-intensity exercise or 75 minutes of vigorous-intensity exercise each week.

Choose exercises that you enjoy: Exercise doesn't have to be a chore. Choose activities that you enjoy, whether it's swimming, hiking, dancing, or playing a sport. When you enjoy your exercise routine, you're more likely to stick with it over the long term.

Incorporate strength training: Strength training can help you build muscle, boost your metabolism, and burn more calories. Aim to include strength training exercises at least two days a week, focusing on all major muscle groups.

Don't rely on exercise alone: While exercise is an important part of weight loss, it's not the only factor. Eating a healthy diet is also essential. Don't rely on exercise alone to help you lose weight.

By combining exercise and healthy eating, you can create a powerful weight loss strategy that will help you achieve your goals more quickly and efficiently. Remember to make exercise a regular part of your routine, choose activities that you enjoy, and fuel your body with healthy foods and plenty of water. With consistency and dedication, you can achieve the results you're looking for.

Chapter 24: Understanding the Importance of Rest and Recovery

When embarking on a weight loss journey, it's easy to fall into the trap of thinking that more is always better. More exercise, less food, and fewer breaks may seem like the best way to achieve your goals quickly, but this approach can actually backfire in the long run. Rest and recovery are crucial components of any successful weight loss plan, and understanding their importance is key to achieving and maintaining a healthy weight.

Why Rest and Recovery Are Important

When you exercise, you create tiny tears in your muscle fibers. These tears are a normal part of the process of building strength and endurance, but they also require time and rest to heal properly. Without sufficient rest and recovery time, your muscles can't repair themselves, which can lead to overuse injuries, fatigue, and decreased performance.

Rest and recovery are also important for your overall health and well-being. Chronic stress and lack of sleep can increase your levels of cortisol, a hormone that can contribute to weight gain and other health problems. Taking time to relax and recharge can help to lower your cortisol levels, improve your sleep quality, and reduce your risk of stress-related illnesses.

How to Incorporate Rest and Recovery into Your Weight Loss Plan

Rest and recovery should be an integral part of your weight loss plan, not an afterthought. Here are some strategies for incorporating rest and recovery into your routine:

Prioritize sleep: Aim for seven to eight hours of sleep per night, and make sure that your sleeping environment is dark, quiet, and cool.

Take rest days: Plan at least one day of rest per week, and consider taking more if you're feeling fatigued or experiencing pain.

Incorporate active recovery: On your rest days, consider low-intensity activities like yoga, stretching, or light walking to help improve circulation and promote recovery.

Listen to your body: If you're feeling sore or fatigued, adjust your workouts accordingly. Don't push through pain or injury, as this can lead to more serious problems down the road.

Practice stress-reducing activities: Incorporate activities like meditation, deep breathing, or journaling into your daily routine to help manage stress levels and improve overall well-being.

By prioritizing rest and recovery, you can ensure that your body is able to heal and repair itself, which can help you to achieve your weight loss goals more effectively and sustainably. Remember, weight loss is a journey, not a race, and taking the time to rest and recover along the way is an essential part of that journey.

Chapter 25: The Role of Sleep in Weight Loss

Sleep is an essential component of a healthy lifestyle, and it plays a crucial role in weight loss. Many people underestimate the importance of getting enough quality sleep when it comes to losing weight, but the truth is that sleep deprivation can have a negative impact on your weight loss efforts.

Lack of sleep can disrupt your body's natural hormonal balance, leading to an increase in appetite and a decrease in metabolism. Studies have shown that people who don't get enough sleep are more likely to overeat and make poor food choices, leading to weight gain.

When you're sleep-deprived, your body produces more of the hormone ghrelin, which stimulates appetite, and less of the hormone leptin, which signals satiety. This can lead to increased hunger and cravings for high-calorie, high-fat foods, which can sabotage your weight loss efforts.

In addition to affecting appetite and metabolism, lack of sleep can also impact your energy levels and motivation to exercise. When you're tired, you may be less likely to engage in physical activity, which can further slow down your weight loss progress.

So how much sleep do you need for optimal weight loss? The National Sleep Foundation recommends that adults get 7-9 hours of sleep per night. However, the quality of your sleep is just as important as the quantity. To improve the quality of your sleep, try to establish a regular sleep routine, avoid caffeine and alcohol before bedtime, and create a comfortable sleep environment.

Getting enough quality sleep is a crucial aspect of a healthy lifestyle and an important factor in weight loss. By prioritizing sleep and making it a priority in your weight loss journey, you can improve your chances of success and achieve your weight loss goals more easily.

Chapter 26: How Stress Affects Weight Loss and Strategies for Managing Stress

Stress is an unavoidable part of life, and it can have a significant impact on your weight loss journey. When you're stressed, your body produces more of the hormone cortisol, which can increase your appetite and cause you to store more fat in your abdomen. This can make it harder to lose weight and maintain a healthy weight over time. Additionally, stress can lead to emotional eating, as people often turn to food for comfort or as a coping mechanism.

Managing stress is crucial for successful weight loss. Here are some strategies for managing stress and staying on track with your weight loss goals:

Practice mindfulness: Mindfulness techniques, such as meditation and deep breathing exercises, can help reduce stress and anxiety. Incorporating these practices into your daily routine can help you stay calm and centered, even during stressful situations.

Exercise regularly: Exercise is a great stress reliever and can help improve your mood. Even a short walk or yoga session can help reduce stress and promote relaxation.

Prioritize self-care: Make time for activities that make you feel good, whether it's taking a bubble bath, reading a book, or spending time with friends and family. Taking care of yourself can help reduce stress and improve your overall well-being.

Get enough sleep: Lack of sleep can contribute to stress and make it harder to manage. Aim for at least 7-8 hours of sleep each night to help reduce stress and improve your mood.

Identify and avoid stress triggers: Take note of situations or people that tend to trigger stress for you, and try to avoid or minimize these triggers as much as possible.

Seek professional help if needed: If you're struggling with chronic stress or anxiety, it's important to seek professional help. A therapist or counselor can help you develop coping strategies and provide support and guidance.

Incorporating stress management techniques into your weight loss journey can help you stay on track and reach your goals. Remember, managing stress is just as important as eating healthy and exercising regularly for successful weight loss.

Chapter 27: The Benefits of a Positive Attitude for Weight Loss

Losing weight is a challenging task that requires dedication, discipline, and commitment. It involves making significant changes to your lifestyle, including your eating habits and physical activity. While the process of shedding pounds may seem daunting, having a positive attitude can make all the difference in your weight loss journey. In this chapter, we will explore the benefits of maintaining a positive attitude for weight loss.

Increases Motivation and Consistency

Having a positive attitude can increase your motivation and help you stay consistent in your weight loss journey. A positive mindset can help you set achievable goals, stay focused on your progress, and keep you motivated to keep going even when you encounter obstacles.

When you have a positive attitude, you're more likely to be optimistic and hopeful about your weight loss journey. This positivity can help you maintain your focus and commitment, leading to consistent effort and progress towards your weight loss goals.

Reduces Stress and Anxiety

Weight loss can be stressful, and it's normal to feel anxious about it. However, a positive attitude can help you manage stress and anxiety more effectively. A positive mindset can help you reframe negative thoughts and focus on the positive aspects of your weight loss journey, which can reduce stress and anxiety.

Reducing stress and anxiety is crucial for weight loss because stress and anxiety can lead to overeating, emotional eating, and other unhealthy behaviors that can sabotage your weight loss efforts.

Improves Self-Esteem and Confidence

A positive attitude can also improve your self-esteem and confidence. When you believe in yourself and your ability to succeed, you're more likely to make healthy choices, stick to your weight loss plan, and achieve your goals.

Furthermore, when you focus on the positive changes you're making, you're more likely to feel good about yourself and your progress. This positive self-image can boost your confidence, making it easier to stay on track with your weight loss goals.

Enhances Physical Health

Maintaining a positive attitude can also have physical health benefits. When you're positive, you're more likely to engage in healthy behaviors, such as eating a balanced diet and exercising regularly. These healthy behaviors can help you lose weight and improve your overall health.

Furthermore, a positive attitude can also improve your immune system, reduce inflammation, and lower your risk of developing chronic diseases such as heart disease and diabetes.

Conclusion

In conclusion, maintaining a positive attitude is crucial for weight loss. It can increase your motivation and consistency, reduce stress and anxiety, improve your self-esteem and confidence, and enhance your physical health. Therefore, it's essential to cultivate a positive mindset and focus on the positive aspects of your weight loss journey. By doing so, you'll be more likely to succeed and achieve your weight loss goals.

Chapter 28: Overcoming Obstacles and Staying Motivated

Losing weight is not an easy task, and there are various obstacles that can hinder your progress. However, overcoming these obstacles is crucial if you want to achieve your weight loss goals. In this chapter, we will explore some common obstacles that people face when trying to lose weight and discuss effective ways to stay motivated.

Identifying Obstacles

One of the first steps to overcoming obstacles is to identify them. Here are some common obstacles that people face when trying to lose weight:

Lack of time: Many people struggle to find the time to exercise or prepare healthy meals because of their busy schedules.

Cravings: Food cravings can be one of the biggest obstacles to losing weight. It can be difficult to resist the temptation of unhealthy snacks and desserts.

Plateaus: Weight loss plateaus can be frustrating and demotivating. You may feel like you are putting in a lot of effort without seeing any results.

Lack of Support: Losing weight can be challenging, especially if you do not have support from friends or family members.

Strategies for Overcoming Obstacles

Once you have identified your obstacles, you can take steps to overcome them. Here are some strategies that can help:

Plan Ahead: Lack of time can be a significant obstacle to weight loss. However, by planning your meals and exercise routine ahead of time, you can ensure that you have enough time to prepare healthy meals and work out.

Practice Mindful Eating: Food cravings can be difficult to overcome, but practicing mindful eating can help. Pay attention to your hunger cues and focus on eating nutrient-dense foods that will keep you satisfied for longer.

Change Things Up: Weight loss plateaus can be frustrating, but changing up your routine can help kickstart your weight loss again. Try a new exercise routine or adjust your calorie intake to break through the plateau.

Find Support: Losing weight can be a lonely journey, but having support from friends or family members can make all the difference. Consider joining a support group or reaching out to a friend who has similar weight loss goals.

Staying Motivated

Motivation is crucial when it comes to losing weight. Here are some tips to help you stay motivated:

Set Realistic Goals: Setting unrealistic goals can lead to disappointment and demotivation. Instead, set small, achievable goals that will help you build momentum.

Track Your Progress: Keeping track of your progress can help you see how far you have come and stay motivated. Consider using a food journal or fitness tracker to monitor your progress.

Celebrate Your Successes: Celebrating your successes, no matter how small they may seem, can help you stay motivated. Treat yourself to a non-food reward, such as a new outfit or a massage, when you reach a milestone.

Practice Self-Care: Taking care of yourself is crucial when it comes to staying motivated. Make time for relaxation and stress-reducing activities, such as meditation or yoga.

Conclusion

Overcoming obstacles and staying motivated are essential when it comes to losing weight. By identifying your obstacles and taking steps to overcome them, you can stay on track towards your weight loss goals. Remember to set realistic goals, track your progress, celebrate your successes, and practice self-care to stay motivated and focused on your weight loss journey.

Chapter 29: Fitting Exercise into a Busy Schedule

Fitting exercise into a busy schedule can be a daunting task, but it is crucial for achieving weight loss goals. Exercise is essential for burning calories, building muscle, and improving overall health. Here are some tips on how to fit exercise into your busy schedule.

Plan Ahead: One of the most important things to do when fitting exercise into a busy schedule is to plan ahead. Schedule a specific time for exercise each day, and make it a priority. Treat exercise like any other important appointment, and don't let other obligations get in the way.

Make it a Habit: Making exercise a habit is another essential step to fitting it into a busy schedule. Once you establish a routine, it becomes easier to find the time and motivation to exercise. Start small and gradually increase the amount of time and intensity of your workouts.

Multi-Task: Look for ways to combine exercise with other tasks. For example, take a walk during your lunch break or use an exercise bike while watching TV. You can also try doing some simple exercises while working at your desk or standing instead of sitting during phone calls.

Prioritize Intensity: When time is limited, prioritize high-intensity exercises that burn more calories in less time. HIIT (High-Intensity Interval Training) workouts are a great option as they require short bursts of intense exercise followed by rest periods.

Find a Workout Buddy: Having a workout buddy can help you stay motivated and committed to your fitness goals. It can also make exercise more enjoyable and fun. Consider asking a friend, coworker, or family member to join you in your workouts.

Incorporate Fitness into your Commute: If you commute to work or school, try incorporating exercise into your commute. Consider walking or cycling to work, or getting off a few stops early on public transportation to get some extra steps in.

Use Technology to Your Advantage: There are plenty of fitness apps and gadgets available that can help you fit exercise into your busy schedule. Consider using a fitness tracker or downloading a workout app to help keep you motivated and on track.

Fitting exercise into a busy schedule can be challenging, but it is possible with some planning, dedication, and creativity. Remember, every little bit counts, so even small amounts of exercise throughout the day can add up and help you achieve your weight loss goals.

Chapter 30: Weight Loss and the Workplace

Losing weight is a challenging task, and it can be particularly difficult when it comes to managing weight loss in the workplace. Many people spend a significant portion of their day at work, which can make it difficult to maintain healthy eating habits and regular exercise routines. In this chapter, we will explore the impact of the workplace on weight loss and provide practical strategies to help you achieve your weight loss goals.

The Impact of the Workplace on Weight Loss

The workplace can have a significant impact on weight loss. Long work hours, sedentary jobs, and access to unhealthy food options can all contribute to weight gain. Additionally, workplace stress and fatigue can make it challenging to stick to a healthy eating plan or find the motivation to exercise.

One of the biggest challenges of losing weight in the workplace is the availability of unhealthy food options. Many workplaces have vending machines or cafeterias that offer unhealthy snacks and meals, which can make it difficult to resist temptation. Additionally, coworkers may bring in treats or participate in food-focused activities, such as potlucks or birthday celebrations, which can lead to overeating.

Long work hours and sedentary jobs can also contribute to weight gain. Sitting for long periods of time can slow down metabolism and increase the risk of obesity, diabetes, and other health problems. Moreover, long work hours can leave little time for exercise or meal planning, making it more challenging to maintain a healthy weight.

Strategies for Weight Loss in the Workplace

Despite the challenges of losing weight in the workplace, there are several strategies that you can use to achieve your weight loss goals. These include:

Pack Your Lunch: Bringing your lunch from home can help you avoid the temptation of unhealthy food options in the workplace. Pack a healthy lunch that includes lean protein, vegetables, and whole grains to keep you feeling full and energized throughout the day.

Keep Healthy Snacks on Hand: Stock your desk or workplace with healthy snacks, such as nuts, fruit, or whole-grain crackers. These snacks can help keep you satisfied between meals and prevent overeating.

Find Opportunities to Move: Look for opportunities to move throughout the day, such as taking the stairs instead of the elevator, going for a walk during your lunch break, or doing some stretches at your desk.

Limit Workplace Treats: While it can be tempting to indulge in workplace treats, it's essential to limit your intake. Consider sharing a treat with a coworker or only having a small portion to satisfy your cravings without overeating.

Set Realistic Goals: Set realistic weight loss goals that take into account your work schedule and responsibilities. Rather than trying to lose a significant amount of weight quickly, aim to lose a pound or two per week through healthy eating and exercise.

Manage Workplace Stress: Stress can make it challenging to stick to a healthy eating plan or find the motivation to exercise. Find healthy ways to manage workplace stress, such as taking breaks throughout the day, practicing mindfulness or meditation, or talking to a supportive coworker or friend.

Conclusion

Weight loss in the workplace can be challenging, but it's not impossible. By taking small steps to improve your eating habits and exercise routine, you can achieve your weight loss goals and improve your overall health and well-being. Remember to be patient and kind to yourself, and seek support from coworkers or a healthcare professional if needed. With dedication and persistence, you can successfully lose weight and improve your health, even in the workplace.

Chapter 31: Avoiding Common Weight Loss Mistakes

Losing weight can be a challenging and daunting task for many people, and unfortunately, it is all too easy to make mistakes that can hinder your progress. To help you on your weight loss journey, it's essential to be aware of common weight loss mistakes and learn how to avoid them.

Not Eating Enough or Skipping Meals

One of the most common weight loss mistakes people make is not eating enough or skipping meals. While it might seem logical to cut back on calories to lose weight, drastically reducing your calorie intake can backfire. Your body needs a certain amount of calories to function correctly, and if you don't consume enough, your metabolism can slow down, making it harder to lose weight. Skipping meals can also lead to overeating later in the day, making it more difficult to stay within your calorie goals.

Instead, focus on eating nutrient-dense foods that will fuel your body and keep you feeling full and satisfied throughout the day. Aim to eat three balanced meals a day with healthy snacks in between if needed.

Not Drinking Enough Water

Drinking enough water is crucial for weight loss, yet it's a mistake that many people make. Water helps to flush toxins from your body, boosts your metabolism, and keeps you feeling full, reducing your chances of overeating.

To avoid this mistake, make it a habit to drink at least 8-10 glasses of water a day. You can also try infusing your water with fruits and herbs to make it more flavorful and enjoyable.

Over-Restricting Certain Foods

Eliminating entire food groups or over-restricting certain foods can make it difficult to stick to a healthy eating plan long-term. Instead, focus on moderation and balance. Allow yourself to enjoy your favorite foods in moderation and find healthier alternatives to your favorite indulgences.

Relying on Fad Diets

Fad diets may promise quick weight loss results, but they often aren't sustainable or healthy in the long run. Many fad diets restrict entire food groups or severely limit your calorie intake, which can lead to nutrient deficiencies and metabolic damage.

Instead of relying on fad diets, focus on making long-term lifestyle changes that promote sustainable weight loss. Aim to eat a balanced diet that includes plenty of fruits, vegetables, whole grains, and lean proteins. Also, make exercise a regular part of your routine to help you burn calories and build muscle.

Not Getting Enough Sleep

Sleep is crucial for overall health and well-being, including weight loss. Lack of sleep can disrupt your hormone levels, making it harder to lose weight and increasing your chances of overeating.

To avoid this mistake, make sure you get enough sleep each night. Aim for 7-8 hours of quality sleep per night and establish a regular sleep routine to help you fall asleep and wake up at the same time each day.

In conclusion, avoiding common weight loss mistakes is crucial for achieving sustainable weight loss. By eating a balanced diet, drinking enough water, getting enough sleep, and avoiding fad diets and over-restricting certain foods, you can achieve your weight loss goals and maintain a healthy lifestyle.

Chapter 32: The Benefits of Tracking Your Food Intake

When it comes to losing weight, one of the most important factors is ensuring that you are consuming fewer calories than you are burning. While exercise can help to increase the number of calories you burn each day, it can be difficult to accurately estimate the number of calories you are consuming through food without tracking your intake.

Tracking your food intake can provide a number of benefits when it comes to losing weight. Here are some of the key advantages:

Helps you stay within your calorie limits

By tracking your food intake, you can ensure that you are staying within your recommended calorie limits. This is especially important if you are trying to lose weight, as consuming too many calories can prevent you from achieving your goals. By tracking your food intake, you can see exactly how many calories you are consuming each day, and adjust your intake as needed to ensure you are staying within your target range.

Identifies problem areas

Tracking your food intake can help you identify problem areas in your diet. For example, you may find that you are consuming too many calories from high-fat foods, or that you are not getting enough protein in your diet. By identifying these problem areas, you can make adjustments to your diet to ensure that you are getting the nutrients you need without consuming too many calories.

Increases awareness

Tracking your food intake can also increase your awareness of what you are eating. Many people consume food without thinking about it, which can lead to overeating and weight gain. By tracking your food intake, you become more mindful of what you are eating, which can help you make better choices and avoid overeating.

Provides motivation

Finally, tracking your food intake can provide motivation when it comes to losing weight. When you see progress over time, it can be incredibly motivating and can help you stay on track. Additionally, tracking your food intake can help you see the impact of your food choices on your weight loss, which can be a powerful motivator to continue making healthy choices.

Overall, tracking your food intake can be an incredibly helpful tool when it comes to losing weight. By providing insight into your calorie intake, identifying problem areas, increasing awareness, and providing motivation, tracking your food intake can help you achieve your weight loss goals and maintain a healthy weight over the long term.

Chapter 33: Healthy and Easy-to-Make Meal and Snack Recipes

When it comes to losing weight, healthy eating plays a crucial role. However, preparing healthy meals can be time-consuming and overwhelming. That's why we have compiled a list of easy-to-make meal and snack recipes that are both delicious and nutritious.

Breakfast: Berry and Yogurt Smoothie Bowl

Ingredients:

1 cup frozen mixed berries

1 banana

1/2 cup Greek yogurt

1/4 cup almond milk

1 tablespoon honey

Toppings: sliced strawberries, blueberries, chia seeds, and granola

Directions:

Combine the frozen mixed berries, banana, Greek yogurt, almond milk, and honey in a blender and blend until smooth.

Pour the mixture into a bowl and add your desired toppings.

Lunch: Chickpea and Avocado Salad

Ingredients:

1 can chickpeas, drained and rinsed

1 avocado, diced

1/2 cup cherry tomatoes, halved

1/4 cup red onion, diced

2 tablespoons olive oil

2 tablespoons lemon juice

Salt and pepper to taste

Directions:

In a large bowl, combine the chickpeas, avocado, cherry tomatoes, and red onion.

Drizzle the olive oil and lemon juice over the top and toss to combine.

Season with salt and pepper to taste.

Dinner: Grilled Chicken with Roasted Vegetables

Ingredients:

4 boneless, skinless chicken breasts

1 red bell pepper, sliced

1 yellow bell pepper, sliced

1 zucchini, sliced

1 red onion, sliced

2 tablespoons olive oil

Salt and pepper to taste

Directions:

Preheat the grill to medium-high heat.

Brush the chicken breasts with olive oil and season with salt and pepper.

Grill the chicken for 6-8 minutes per side, or until cooked through.

Meanwhile, preheat the oven to 400°F.

Arrange the sliced vegetables on a baking sheet and drizzle with olive oil.

Roast the vegetables for 15-20 minutes, or until tender.

Chapter 34: Identifying and Overcoming Self-Sabotaging Behaviors

When it comes to losing weight, one of the biggest obstacles that many people face is self-sabotage. Self-sabotaging behaviors can take many forms, from indulging in unhealthy foods to avoiding exercise to making excuses for not sticking to a healthy eating plan.

Identifying these self-sabotaging behaviors is the first step in overcoming them. Here are some common examples:

Negative self-talk: This can include telling yourself that you're not capable of losing weight, or that you'll never be able to stick to a healthy eating plan. Negative self-talk can be very destructive and can make it difficult to achieve your weight loss goals.

Emotional eating: This is when you turn to food as a way to deal with emotions such as stress, anxiety, or sadness. Emotional eating can lead to overeating and can make it difficult to maintain a healthy weight.

Lack of planning: If you don't plan ahead and have healthy food options available, it can be easy to fall into the trap of grabbing unhealthy snacks or fast food on the go.

All-or-nothing thinking: This is when you believe that you have to be perfect with your eating and exercise habits, and if you slip up even once, you've failed. This kind of thinking can be very damaging and can make it difficult to get back on track after a setback.

Once you've identified these self-sabotaging behaviors, the next step is to start working on overcoming them. Here are some strategies that can help:

Replace negative self-talk with positive affirmations: Instead of telling yourself that you can't do something, tell yourself that you're capable and strong. Focus on your successes and celebrate your accomplishments, no matter how small they may seem.

Find healthier ways to deal with emotions: Instead of turning to food when you're feeling stressed or sad, try going for a walk, practicing deep breathing, or calling a friend for support.

Plan ahead: Take some time each week to plan out your meals and snacks, and make sure you have healthy options on hand. This will make it easier to stick to a healthy eating plan and avoid unhealthy temptations.

Practice moderation: Remember that it's okay to indulge in your favorite foods once in a while. The key is to practice moderation and balance, and to get back on track with healthy habits as soon as possible.

By identifying and overcoming self-sabotaging behaviors, you can set yourself up for success on your weight loss journey. Remember that change takes time, and it's okay to make mistakes along the way. The important thing is to keep moving forward, one healthy choice at a time.

Chapter 35: The Benefits of Meditation and Mindfulness for Weight Loss

When it comes to weight loss, most people focus on diet and exercise as the primary strategies. However, meditation and mindfulness can also be powerful tools in achieving weight loss goals. Here are some benefits of incorporating meditation and mindfulness into your weight loss plan:

Reducing Stress and Emotional Eating

Stress and emotional eating are common reasons for overeating and weight gain. Meditation and mindfulness can help reduce stress levels by calming the mind and promoting relaxation. When you are less stressed, you are less likely to turn to food for comfort or to cope with negative emotions.

Improving Self-Awareness and Self-Control

Mindfulness practices involve paying attention to the present moment without judgment. By practicing mindfulness during meals and snacks, you can become more aware of your hunger and satiety cues. This can help you make more conscious decisions about when and how much to eat, leading to better portion control and fewer instances of overeating.

Boosting Metabolism

Meditation and mindfulness have been shown to help regulate the body's stress response and balance hormones such as cortisol, which can affect metabolism. By reducing stress and promoting relaxation, meditation and mindfulness may help boost your metabolism and support weight loss.

Supporting Healthy Habits

Meditation and mindfulness can help you cultivate a sense of mindfulness and awareness that extends beyond meal times. This can lead to a greater overall sense of self-care, making it easier to prioritize healthy habits like regular exercise and getting enough sleep.

Enhancing Body Awareness

Meditation and mindfulness can also help you become more attuned to your body's physical sensations, including hunger and fullness. This can help you differentiate between true hunger and emotional cravings, making it easier to make healthier food choices.

Incorporating meditation and mindfulness into your weight loss plan can be as simple as taking a few deep breaths before meals or practicing a short guided meditation each day. By reducing stress and increasing self-awareness, meditation and mindfulness can help support your weight loss goals and promote a healthier relationship with food and your body.

Chapter 36: Weight Loss and Hormones

Losing weight can be a challenge for many people, and while diet and exercise are important factors, hormones also play a significant role. Hormones are chemical messengers in the body that regulate a wide range of functions, including metabolism, appetite, and energy expenditure. Here, we will explore some of the key hormones involved in weight loss and how they can impact your weight loss journey.

Leptin

Leptin is a hormone produced by fat cells that regulates appetite and metabolism. It sends signals to the brain to reduce hunger and increase energy expenditure, helping to maintain a healthy weight. However, in overweight or obese individuals, leptin resistance can occur, meaning the brain doesn't respond to leptin's signals to reduce hunger or increase metabolism. This can result in increased appetite and decreased energy expenditure, making weight loss more difficult.

To combat leptin resistance, it's important to focus on a healthy diet that includes plenty of fiber, protein, and healthy fats. These nutrients can help regulate hormones and improve leptin sensitivity. Additionally, regular exercise can also improve leptin sensitivity, helping to reduce hunger and promote weight loss.

Ghrelin

Ghrelin is a hormone produced by the stomach that stimulates appetite. It sends signals to the brain to increase hunger, making it difficult to maintain a healthy weight. However, ghrelin levels can be reduced through regular exercise and sleep. Exercise has been shown to decrease ghrelin levels, while getting enough sleep can help regulate hormone levels and reduce hunger.

Insulin

Insulin is a hormone produced by the pancreas that regulates blood sugar levels. It helps the body convert glucose into energy, but when there's too much glucose in the bloodstream, the body stores it as fat. Therefore, it's important to regulate insulin levels through a healthy diet that includes plenty of complex carbohydrates, fiber, and protein. Additionally, exercise can also help regulate insulin levels and promote weight loss.

Cortisol

Cortisol is a hormone produced by the adrenal glands that regulates stress response. When cortisol levels are high, it can increase appetite and promote the storage of fat in the abdominal area. Therefore, it's important to manage stress levels through techniques like meditation, yoga, or other stress-reducing activities. Getting enough sleep and exercise can also help reduce cortisol levels and promote weight loss.

In conclusion, hormones play a significant role in weight loss, and understanding how they work can help you reach your weight loss goals. Focus on a healthy diet that includes plenty of fiber, protein, and healthy fats, as well as regular exercise and stress-reducing activities. By regulating your hormones, you can improve your metabolism, reduce hunger, and promote weight loss.

Chapter 37: The Dangers of Crash Dieting and Fad Diets

When it comes to losing weight, there are a plethora of diets and weight loss programs that promise quick and easy results. However, many of these diets are not only ineffective but also dangerous to one's health. In this chapter, we will delve into the dangers of crash dieting and fad diets.

Crash Dieting: The Quick Fix that Doesn't Last

Crash dieting is a term used to describe a short-term, drastic reduction in calorie intake to achieve rapid weight loss. These diets often eliminate entire food groups and severely restrict calories, which can lead to rapid weight loss in a short amount of time. However, crash diets are not sustainable, and the weight loss achieved is often short-lived. As soon as you return to your normal eating habits, the weight you lost will quickly return.

One of the major dangers of crash dieting is that it can lead to malnutrition. When you drastically reduce your calorie intake, your body doesn't get the nutrients it needs to function properly. This can result in fatigue, weakness, dizziness, and even fainting.

Another danger of crash dieting is that it can slow down your metabolism. When you drastically reduce your calorie intake, your body goes into starvation mode and begins to conserve energy by slowing down your metabolism. This means that when you return to your normal eating habits, your body will burn fewer calories, making it more difficult to lose weight.

Fad Diets: The False Promises that Don't Deliver

Fad diets are diets that promise quick weight loss through unconventional methods. These diets often eliminate entire food groups or require you to consume large amounts of a specific food. While fad diets may seem appealing due to their promises of quick weight loss, they are often unhealthy and ineffective.

One of the biggest dangers of fad diets is that they can lead to nutrient deficiencies. Eliminating entire food groups can deprive your body of essential nutrients, leading to malnutrition and other health problems.

Another danger of fad diets is that they can be unsustainable. Many fad diets are too restrictive and difficult to follow long-term, leading to weight regain once you return to your normal eating habits.

Additionally, many fad diets are not backed by scientific evidence and can be harmful to your health. For example, the keto diet, which requires you to consume large amounts of fat and severely restrict carbohydrates, can lead to an increase in cholesterol levels and may increase your risk of heart disease.

The Bottom Line

Crash dieting and fad diets may promise quick weight loss, but they are not sustainable and can be harmful to your health. Instead of looking for a quick fix, focus on making small, sustainable changes to your diet and lifestyle. Eat a balanced diet that includes a variety of nutrient-dense foods, and engage in regular physical activity. Remember, slow and steady progress is the key to long-term weight loss success.

Chapter 38: The Benefits of Gradual and Sustainable Weight Loss

Losing weight is a journey, and it can be tempting to try to rush to the finish line. But as the saying goes, slow and steady wins the race. Gradual and sustainable weight loss is not only more effective, but it also has numerous benefits for your health and well-being. In this chapter, we'll explore why slow and steady wins the weight loss race.

Lower Risk of Regaining Weight

One of the most significant benefits of gradual and sustainable weight loss is that it is more likely to be maintained in the long run. Rapid weight loss often leads to a rebound effect, where people regain the weight they lost and sometimes even more. This is because quick weight loss typically involves drastic calorie restriction and unsustainable lifestyle changes. When you lose weight gradually and sustainably, you give your body time to adjust to new habits, and you are more likely to make permanent changes to your lifestyle that support weight maintenance.

Improved Health Markers

Losing weight gradually and sustainably can also lead to significant improvements in health markers. For example, research has shown that losing just 5-10% of your body weight can lower your risk of developing type 2 diabetes, high blood pressure, and heart disease. Losing weight gradually also reduces the risk of gallbladder disease and certain types of cancer, including breast, colon, and prostate cancer. Additionally, losing weight slowly and sustainably can lead to improvements in cholesterol levels, blood sugar levels, and insulin sensitivity.

Better Mental Health

Losing weight can be stressful, but it can also have a positive impact on your mental health. Gradual and sustainable weight loss can improve your self-esteem, reduce stress and anxiety, and improve your overall mood. This is because when you lose weight slowly and sustainably, you are more likely to make lifestyle changes that you enjoy and that fit into your daily routine. This can lead to a sense of accomplishment and increased confidence, which can have a positive impact on your mental well-being.

More Sustainable Lifestyle Changes

When you lose weight gradually and sustainably, you are more likely to make lifestyle changes that are sustainable in the long run. This means that you are less likely to feel deprived, and you are more likely to enjoy the changes you have made. For example, if you enjoy walking, you are more likely to continue walking regularly than if you force yourself to do high-intensity interval training every day. This can help you maintain your weight loss in the long run and enjoy a healthier lifestyle overall.

In conclusion, gradual and sustainable weight loss is more effective and has numerous benefits for your health and well-being. By losing weight slowly and sustainably, you can reduce your risk of regaining weight, improve your health markers, boost your mental health, and make lifestyle changes that are more sustainable in the long run. So don't rush to the finish line; instead, take your time and enjoy the journey.

Chapter 39: Mind-Body Connection for Weight Loss

The mind and body are interconnected in more ways than we often realize. Our thoughts, emotions, and beliefs can all have an impact on our physical health and well-being, including our ability to lose weight. By understanding the mind-body connection, we can take a more holistic approach to weight loss that focuses on both our mental and physical health.

One of the key ways that the mind and body are connected in relation to weight loss is through stress. When we experience stress, our bodies release the hormone cortisol, which can lead to increased appetite, cravings for unhealthy foods, and weight gain. Additionally, stress can also lead to emotional eating, which can further exacerbate the problem.

To combat this, it's important to find ways to manage stress in our lives. This might include practicing mindfulness or meditation, getting regular exercise, or engaging in other stress-relieving activities like yoga or tai chi. By reducing stress levels, we can help our bodies function more optimally, which can lead to better weight loss results.

Another way that the mind-body connection impacts weight loss is through our beliefs and attitudes towards food and exercise. If we have negative beliefs or a poor self-image when it comes to our bodies, it can be difficult to stay motivated and committed to healthy habits. On the other hand, if we have a positive mindset and a sense of self-efficacy, we are more likely to stick to our goals and achieve success.

To cultivate a positive mindset, it's important to focus on self-compassion and self-care. This might involve practicing positive self-talk, surrounding ourselves with supportive friends and family members, or seeking out professional help if needed. By nurturing a positive attitude towards ourselves and our bodies, we can create a more sustainable and fulfilling weight loss journey.

Finally, the mind-body connection can also impact weight loss through our sleeping habits. Research has shown that inadequate sleep can lead to a host of negative health outcomes, including weight gain and obesity. This is because sleep deprivation can disrupt hormone levels and increase cravings for unhealthy foods.

To ensure that we are getting enough restful sleep, it's important to establish a regular sleep routine and create a relaxing environment for sleep. This might include avoiding electronic devices before bedtime, creating a comfortable sleeping space, and sticking to a consistent sleep schedule. By prioritizing our sleep, we can improve our overall health and support our weight loss goals.

In conclusion, the mind-body connection plays a critical role in our ability to lose weight and achieve our health goals. By addressing stress, cultivating a positive mindset, and prioritizing sleep, we can create a more holistic approach to weight loss that supports both our physical and mental well-being.

Chapter 40: How to Stay Motivated When Progress Slows

When it comes to losing weight, progress can often be slow and challenging, leading to a loss of motivation. However, maintaining your motivation during these challenging times is key to achieving your weight loss goals. Here are some strategies to help you stay motivated when progress slows down.

Focus on Your Why: Reconnect with your reasons for wanting to lose weight. Is it to improve your health, feel more confident, or be more active with your family?

Remind yourself of these reasons regularly and use them as a source of motivation to keep going.

Celebrate Small Wins: It's easy to get discouraged when progress is slow, but it's important to recognize and celebrate your small wins along the way. Did you make healthier food choices today? Did you increase the amount of exercise you did this week? Celebrate these accomplishments and use them to fuel your motivation.

Change Up Your Routine: If progress has slowed down, it may be time to change up your routine. Try a new workout, switch up your meal plan, or challenge yourself to try something new. This can help reignite your motivation and give you a fresh perspective on your weight loss journey.

Seek Support: Having a support system can be incredibly helpful when progress slows down. Reach out to friends or family members who can offer encouragement and support, or consider joining a weight loss support group. Knowing that you have people cheering you on can be a powerful motivator.

Practice Self-Care: Taking care of yourself can help you stay motivated during challenging times. Make time for activities that you enjoy, such as reading, listening to music, or taking a relaxing bath. Also, prioritize getting enough sleep, drinking plenty of water, and eating nutritious foods to help you feel your best.

Remember that Progress Takes Time: It's important to remember that progress takes time, and weight loss is not a linear journey. There will be ups and downs along the way, and that's okay. Be patient with yourself and trust the process. Stay focused on your goals and stay motivated, even when progress is slow.

By following these strategies, you can stay motivated during challenging times and continue making progress towards your weight loss goals. Remember to stay positive, stay committed, and celebrate your small wins along the way.

Chapter 41: The Benefits of Weight Loss for Overall Health

Weight loss is a common goal for many people, and for good reason. It has numerous benefits for overall health that extend far beyond just physical appearance. In fact, shedding excess pounds can improve nearly every aspect of your health, from your cardiovascular system to your mental well-being.

One of the primary benefits of weight loss is a reduction in the risk of chronic diseases. Obesity is a major risk factor for conditions such as heart disease, stroke, type 2 diabetes, and certain cancers. By losing weight, you can lower your risk of developing these conditions and improve your overall health outcomes.

Weight loss can also improve cardiovascular health. Carrying excess weight places a significant strain on the heart, increasing the risk of heart disease and stroke. Losing even a small amount of weight can help to reduce blood pressure, lower cholesterol levels, and improve heart function. This can lead to a lower risk of heart disease and other cardiovascular problems.

Another benefit of weight loss is improved mobility and joint health. Carrying extra weight puts a strain on your joints, particularly your knees, hips, and back. This can lead to pain and mobility issues that limit your ability to participate in physical activity. Losing weight can reduce the strain on your joints, improving mobility and reducing the risk of joint-related problems.

Weight loss can also improve sleep quality. Obese individuals are more likely to suffer from sleep apnea and other sleep-related disorders, which can have negative impacts on overall health. Losing weight can help to reduce the severity of these conditions and improve sleep quality, leading to better overall health outcomes.

In addition to physical health benefits, weight loss can also have a positive impact on mental health. Obesity has been linked to an increased risk of depression, anxiety, and other mental health disorders. Losing weight can improve self-esteem and confidence, leading to better mental health outcomes.

Finally, weight loss can improve overall quality of life. By reducing the risk of chronic diseases, improving mobility and joint health, and enhancing mental well-being, weight loss can lead to a better quality of life. It can also improve energy levels, making it easier to participate in physical activity and enjoy daily activities.

In conclusion, weight loss has numerous benefits for overall health. It can reduce the risk of chronic diseases, improve cardiovascular health, enhance mobility and joint health, improve sleep quality, enhance mental well-being, and improve overall quality of life. If you are looking to improve your health, losing weight may be a great place to start.

Chapter 42: Coping with Setbacks and Weight Loss Plateaus

Losing weight can be a challenging journey that requires patience, determination, and perseverance. While the initial stages of weight loss may be motivating and exciting, it's common to experience setbacks and plateaus that can be frustrating and demotivating. In this chapter, we will explore some practical strategies that can help you cope with setbacks and weight loss plateaus and stay on track with your weight loss goals.

Understanding Setbacks and Plateaus

Before diving into the coping strategies, it's essential to understand what setbacks and weight loss plateaus are and why they occur. A setback is a sudden interruption or reversal of progress towards your weight loss goals. It can be caused by various factors such as stress, illness, injury, or emotional eating. On the other hand, a weight loss plateau is a period of time where you stop losing weight despite following your diet and exercise plan. Plateaus can be caused by various factors such as changes in metabolism, water retention, or the body adapting to your exercise routine.

Coping Strategies

Reevaluate Your Goals and Plan: When faced with setbacks or plateaus, it's essential to revisit your weight loss goals and evaluate your plan. Ask yourself if your goals are realistic and achievable, and if your current plan is effective. Consider making adjustments to your diet and exercise plan, such as changing your calorie intake, adding strength training, or trying a new workout routine.

Stay Positive and Motivated: It's natural to feel demotivated and frustrated when faced with setbacks or plateaus, but it's essential to stay positive and motivated.

Remind yourself of the progress you've made so far and focus on the small victories. Surround yourself with positive influences, such as supportive friends and family or a weight loss support group.

Practice Mindful Eating: Mindful eating can help you stay on track with your weight loss goals by reducing emotional eating and promoting healthy eating habits. Practice mindful eating by eating slowly, chewing your food thoroughly, and focusing on the flavors and textures of your food. Avoid eating in front of the TV or computer, and instead, sit at a table and savor your meals.

Track Your Progress: Tracking your progress can help you stay accountable and motivated. Keep a food diary to track your calorie intake and monitor your weight loss progress. Use a fitness tracker or app to track your exercise routine and monitor your daily activity level.

Celebrate Non-Scale Victories: Non-scale victories are accomplishments that don't involve a number on the scale. Celebrate these victories, such as fitting into a smaller size of clothes, running a mile without stopping, or completing a challenging workout. Non-scale victories can help you stay motivated and remind you of the progress you've made.

In conclusion, setbacks and weight loss plateaus are common on the weight loss journey. However, with the right mindset and strategies, you can cope with these challenges and stay on track with your weight loss goals. Remember to stay positive, reevaluate your goals and plan, practice mindful eating, track your progress, and celebrate non-scale victories. With these strategies in mind, you can overcome setbacks and plateaus and achieve your weight loss goals.

Chapter 43: The Importance of Strength Training for Weight Loss

When most people think about losing weight, they often focus solely on cardio workouts and reducing their caloric intake. However, strength training is an essential component of any effective weight loss program.

Strength training, also known as resistance training or weight lifting, involves using weights or other forms of resistance to strengthen and tone your muscles. While cardio workouts like running and cycling are great for burning calories and improving cardiovascular health, strength training offers a unique set of benefits that can help you lose weight and keep it off.

First and foremost, strength training helps to increase your muscle mass. This is important because muscle tissue is metabolically active, meaning it burns more calories at rest than fat tissue. By increasing your muscle mass, you'll be able to burn more calories throughout the day, even when you're not working out.

In addition to increasing your metabolism, strength training can also help you to burn more calories during your workouts. When you engage in strength training, you're challenging your muscles to lift heavy weights or perform difficult movements. This places a significant demand on your body, which causes you to burn more calories than you would during a lower-intensity workout.

Another benefit of strength training is that it can help you to preserve your muscle mass while you're losing weight. When you're in a calorie deficit, your body may turn to your muscle tissue for energy. However, by engaging in strength training, you're sending a signal to your body that your muscles are important and that you need them to stay strong. This can help to prevent muscle loss and preserve your metabolism as you continue to lose weight.

Strength training can also help to improve your overall body composition. While losing weight is important, what you really want to do is lose fat and maintain or even increase your muscle mass. By incorporating strength training into your weight loss program, you'll be able to achieve a leaner, more toned physique.

Finally, strength training can help to improve your overall health and well-being. Studies have shown that strength training can help to reduce your risk of chronic diseases like heart disease, diabetes, and osteoporosis. It can also improve your balance, coordination, and flexibility, which can help you to stay active and independent as you age.

In conclusion, strength training is an essential component of any effective weight loss program. By increasing your muscle mass, burning more calories, preserving your muscle mass, improving your body composition, and improving your overall health and well-being, strength training can help you to achieve your weight loss goals and maintain a healthy lifestyle for years to come.

Chapter 44: Avoiding Common Exercise Mistakes

Exercise is an essential part of any weight loss journey, but it's important to exercise correctly to avoid injury and maximize results. Unfortunately, many people make common exercise mistakes that hinder their progress. In this chapter, we will discuss some of the most common exercise mistakes and how to avoid them.

Mistake #1: Skipping Warm-Up and Cool-Down

One of the most common exercise mistakes is skipping the warm-up and cool-down. A proper warm-up prepares your body for exercise by increasing blood flow to your muscles and joints, while a cool-down helps your body recover and prevent muscle soreness.

To avoid this mistake, take 5-10 minutes to warm up before exercising. This can include dynamic stretches, light cardio, or foam rolling. Similarly, take 5-10 minutes to cool down after exercise by doing static stretches or low-intensity movements.

Mistake #2: Overtraining

Another common exercise mistake is overtraining. While it's essential to challenge your body during exercise, too much exercise can lead to injury and burnout. Overtraining can also lead to a plateau in weight loss progress.

To avoid overtraining, it's important to rest and recover between workouts. Aim to exercise 3-4 times per week, allowing for at least one day of rest between workouts. You can also incorporate active recovery days, such as yoga or a light walk.

Mistake #3: Poor Form

Proper form is essential to prevent injury and maximize results. Poor form can also lead to muscle imbalances and decreased effectiveness of the exercise.

To avoid poor form, start with lighter weights and focus on technique. Seek guidance from a personal trainer or watch instructional videos to ensure you're performing exercises correctly. Remember to engage your core and maintain good posture throughout each exercise.

Mistake #4: Focusing on One Muscle Group

Many people make the mistake of focusing on one muscle group, neglecting other areas of their body. This can lead to muscle imbalances, which can lead to injury and decreased effectiveness of the exercise.

To avoid this mistake, incorporate exercises that target different muscle groups into your workout routine. This can include compound exercises such as squats, lunges, and push-ups that work multiple muscle groups at once.

Mistake #5: Not Pushing Yourself

While it's important to avoid overtraining, it's also essential to challenge yourself during exercise. Many people make the mistake of not pushing themselves enough, leading to a plateau in weight loss progress.

To avoid this mistake, gradually increase the intensity and duration of your workouts. This can include adding more weight, increasing the number of repetitions, or decreasing rest time between sets. Remember to listen to your body and avoid pushing yourself too hard.

In conclusion, exercise is a crucial part of any weight loss journey. However, it's important to exercise correctly to avoid injury and maximize results. By avoiding these common exercise mistakes, you can achieve your weight loss goals safely and effectively.

Chapter 45: The Benefits of Meal Planning and Preparation for Weight Loss

Meal planning and preparation can be incredibly beneficial for weight loss efforts. It is often said that weight loss is 80% diet and 20% exercise, meaning that what you eat is more important than how much you move. By planning and preparing your meals in advance, you can make sure that you are eating healthy, balanced meals that are designed to help you lose weight.

Here are just a few of the benefits of meal planning and preparation for weight loss:

You Can Control Your Portion Sizes

One of the biggest challenges when it comes to losing weight is controlling your portion sizes. When you eat out or grab food on the go, it can be difficult to know how much you are actually eating. However, when you plan and prepare your meals at home, you have complete control over the amount of food you are consuming. This can help you to avoid overeating and stay within your calorie goals.

You Can Make Healthier Choices

When you plan your meals in advance, you have the opportunity to make healthier choices. You can choose whole, unprocessed foods that are rich in nutrients and low in calories. You can also avoid unhealthy ingredients like added sugars and saturated fats. By making these healthier choices, you can fuel your body with the nutrients it needs to function properly while also creating a calorie deficit that will help you lose weight.

You Can Save Time and Money

Meal planning and preparation can actually save you time and money in the long run. When you plan your meals in advance, you can buy ingredients in bulk and avoid last-minute trips to the grocery store. You can also cook in batches and freeze meals for later, which can save you time on busy weeknights. By cooking at home instead of eating out, you can also save money on expensive restaurant meals.

You Can Reduce Stress

Trying to figure out what to eat for each meal can be stressful and time-consuming. By planning your meals in advance, you can eliminate the stress of decision-making and ensure that you always have a healthy, satisfying meal on hand. This can also help to reduce the temptation to grab unhealthy snacks or fast food when you are hungry and in a rush.

You Can Stay on Track with Your Goals

Finally, meal planning and preparation can help you to stay on track with your weight loss goals. By knowing what you are going to eat in advance, you can avoid making impulsive decisions that could derail your progress. You can also monitor your calorie intake and make adjustments as needed to ensure that you are staying within your daily goals.

In conclusion, meal planning and preparation can be a powerful tool for weight loss. By taking the time to plan your meals in advance and prepare them at home, you can control your portion sizes, make healthier choices, save time and money, reduce stress, and stay on track with your goals. So if you are looking to lose weight, consider giving meal planning and preparation a try!

Chapter 46: Incorporating Mindful Movement into Your Daily Routine

If you're trying to lose weight, you might think that the key is simply to exercise more and eat less. However, there's a more holistic approach to weight loss that involves taking care of your mind and body in a way that encourages a healthy lifestyle.

One effective way to do this is by incorporating mindful movement into your daily routine. Mindful movement refers to any physical activity that is done with intention and awareness of the body's sensations, breathing, and thoughts. Here are some tips for incorporating mindful movement into your daily routine:

Start small: You don't have to run a marathon or join a gym to start incorporating mindful movement into your daily routine. Start by taking a short walk around your block or doing some simple stretches in the morning. As you get more comfortable with these small movements, you can gradually increase the intensity and duration of your exercises.

Focus on your breath: As you move your body, pay attention to your breath. Take slow, deep breaths and focus on the sensations in your body as you inhale and exhale. This will help you stay present in the moment and avoid getting lost in thoughts about the past or future.

Set an intention: Before you start your exercise, set an intention for what you want to get out of it. This might be something as simple as "I want to feel more energized today" or "I want to improve my flexibility." Setting an intention can help you stay motivated and focused on your goals.

Choose activities that you enjoy: Mindful movement doesn't have to be a chore. Choose activities that you genuinely enjoy, whether it's dancing, hiking, yoga, or swimming. When you're having fun, you'll be more likely to stick with your exercise routine.

Be patient with yourself: Mindful movement is a practice, not a quick fix. It takes time to develop a mindful approach to exercise, so be patient with yourself and celebrate small victories along the way. Remember that every time you move your body with intention and awareness, you're making progress towards a healthier, happier you.

Incorporating mindful movement into your daily routine can be a powerful tool for weight loss and overall wellbeing. By taking care of your mind and body through intentional physical activity, you'll not only see physical changes but also experience mental and emotional benefits that will help you maintain a healthy lifestyle.

Chapter 47: The Dangers of Yo-Yo Dieting and Quick Fixes

If you're like most people, you've probably tried a variety of diets over the years, some of which may have promised quick and dramatic weight loss. While it's tempting to want a fast solution to your weight loss struggles, these quick fixes can actually do more harm than good.

Yo-yo dieting, also known as weight cycling, is the practice of losing weight quickly, only to gain it back again just as quickly. This cycle of weight loss and weight gain can be detrimental to your health in several ways.

First and foremost, yo-yo dieting can be hard on your heart. Losing and gaining weight repeatedly can increase your risk of heart disease and high blood pressure, both of which can be life-threatening. Additionally, yo-yo dieting can make it more difficult for you to lose weight in the long term, as your body may become resistant to weight loss efforts over time.

Another danger of quick fixes and yo-yo dieting is that they often involve restrictive eating patterns that can deprive your body of essential nutrients. Many fad diets are low in calories, protein, and healthy fats, which can lead to muscle loss, fatigue, and even malnutrition.

Moreover, quick fixes may encourage you to rely on supplements, meal replacements, or other artificial products to help you lose weight. While these products may help you drop a few pounds in the short term, they are not sustainable or healthy in the long term. These products often contain chemicals, preservatives, and other additives that can be harmful to your health.

Finally, quick fixes and yo-yo dieting can take a toll on your mental health as well. Constantly obsessing over your weight and appearance can lead to anxiety, depression, and poor self-esteem. These negative feelings can create a vicious cycle of emotional eating and further weight gain.

So, what's the solution? Instead of focusing on quick fixes and yo-yo dieting, it's important to adopt a healthy, sustainable lifestyle that includes regular exercise, whole foods, and balanced meals. By making small, gradual changes to your habits over time, you can achieve and maintain a healthy weight without compromising your health or well-being.

In conclusion, the dangers of yo-yo dieting and quick fixes far outweigh any potential benefits. By avoiding fad diets and instead focusing on healthy, sustainable habits, you can achieve your weight loss goals while protecting your health and well-being.

Chapter 48: The Benefits of Working with a Professional for Weight Loss

Losing weight is never easy, and sometimes it can feel like an uphill battle. With so much conflicting information out there about what works and what doesn't, it's easy to get confused and overwhelmed. That's why working with a professional can be a game-changer when it comes to achieving your weight loss goals.

In this chapter, we'll discuss the benefits of working with a professional for weight loss and explore the different types of professionals who can help you along your weight loss journey.

Benefit #1: Personalized Plan

One of the biggest benefits of working with a professional for weight loss is the personalized plan they can create for you. Everyone's body is different, and what works for one person may not work for another. A professional can take into account your specific needs and goals and create a plan that is tailored to you. This can help you achieve better results than following a one-size-fits-all approach.

Benefit #2: Accountability and Support

Another benefit of working with a professional is the accountability and support they can provide. Losing weight can be a lonely journey, and having someone to support you and hold you accountable can make all the difference. A professional can help keep you motivated, track your progress, and provide guidance and encouragement when you need it.

Benefit #3: Expertise and Knowledge

Weight loss can be complicated, and there's a lot to know about nutrition, exercise, and overall health. Working with a professional gives you access to their expertise and knowledge. They can help you navigate the complexities of weight loss and provide insights and advice that you may not have considered on your own.

Types of Professionals

Now that we've discussed the benefits of working with a professional for weight loss, let's take a look at the different types of professionals who can help you along the way.

Registered Dietitian

A registered dietitian is a healthcare professional who specializes in nutrition. They can create a personalized meal plan for you, offer guidance on portion control and healthy eating habits, and help you navigate any dietary restrictions or food allergies.

Personal Trainer

A personal trainer is a fitness professional who can create a workout plan tailored to your needs and goals. They can help you build muscle, increase endurance, and improve your overall fitness level.

Health Coach

A health coach is a professional who can provide guidance and support in all areas of health and wellness, including weight loss. They can help you set goals, create a plan, and provide accountability and support along the way.

Bariatric Surgeon

In some cases, weight loss surgery may be the best option for achieving significant weight loss. A bariatric surgeon can provide guidance on the different types of weight loss surgery available and help you determine if it's the right choice for you.

Conclusion

Working with a professional for weight loss can be a game-changer. They can provide a personalized plan, accountability and support, and expertise and knowledge to help you achieve your goals. Whether you choose to work with a registered dietitian, personal trainer, health coach, or bariatric surgeon, the benefits of working with a professional are clear. So why not give it a try and see how it can help you on your weight loss journey?

Chapter 49: How to Stay on Track During Holidays and Special Occasions

Staying on track with your weight loss journey during holidays and special occasions can be a challenge, but it's not impossible. These events often come with a plethora of food choices, and it can be tempting to indulge in everything that's offered. However, with a little bit of planning and preparation, you can stay on track and continue to make progress towards your weight loss goals.

Here are some tips on how to stay on track during holidays and special occasions:

Plan Ahead

Before the event, take some time to plan your meals and snacks for the day. Look at the menu or ask the host what will be served and decide what you'll eat ahead of time. This way, you won't be tempted to make impulsive choices at the last minute.

Eat a Healthy Breakfast

Start your day with a healthy and filling breakfast. This will help you stay full for longer and avoid overeating later on. Some great options include oatmeal with fruit, eggs and whole wheat toast, or a smoothie with protein powder.

Don't Arrive Hungry

Never arrive at an event feeling ravenous, as this will make it harder to resist temptation. Eat a small snack before leaving home, such as an apple or a handful of almonds, to help curb your hunger.

Watch Your Portions

It's okay to indulge in your favorite treats, but it's important to watch your portions. Stick to small servings and savor every bite.

Fill Up on Veggies

Make sure to include plenty of vegetables on your plate. They're low in calories and high in fiber, which will help you feel full and satisfied.

Stay Hydrated

Drink plenty of water throughout the day to help you stay hydrated and avoid overeating. Avoid sugary drinks like soda or alcohol, which can be high in calories.

Stay Active

Even if you can't stick to your usual exercise routine, try to stay active during the event. Take a walk after your meal, dance to some music, or play a game with family and friends.

Don't Beat Yourself Up

If you slip up and indulge a little too much, don't beat yourself up. One meal or one event won't derail your progress. Just get back on track the next day and continue with your healthy habits.

Staying on track during holidays and special occasions may be challenging, but it's possible with the right mindset and preparation. Remember to plan ahead, watch your portions, and stay active. Most importantly, don't forget to enjoy yourself and have fun!

Chapter 50: The Role of Genetics in Weight Loss

When it comes to weight loss, many factors come into play. Diet, exercise, lifestyle, and genetics all play a role in determining an individual's ability to shed excess weight. While some people can easily lose weight by making simple changes to their diet and exercise routine, others may struggle despite their best efforts. In this chapter, we will explore the role of genetics in weight loss and what it means for individuals looking to lose weight.

The Genetics of Weight

Genetics plays a significant role in an individual's weight. Studies have shown that up to 70% of an individual's weight is determined by genetics, with the remaining 30% being influenced by lifestyle factors such as diet and exercise. Several genes are responsible for regulating body weight, including those that control hunger, metabolism, and fat storage.

One of the most well-known genes linked to obesity is the FTO gene. This gene has been linked to an increased risk of obesity in individuals who carry specific variations of the gene. Another gene linked to weight gain is the MC4R gene, which regulates hunger and energy expenditure. Variations of this gene have been shown to increase the risk of obesity in some individuals.

How Genetics Affects Weight Loss

While genetics can play a significant role in weight gain, it can also affect an individual's ability to lose weight. Some individuals may find it more challenging to lose weight than others due to genetic factors. For example, individuals who carry specific variations of the FTO gene may find it more challenging to lose weight than those who do not carry these variations.

Additionally, genetics can influence an individual's response to different types of diets and exercise. Some people may respond better to a low-carb diet, while others may see better results with a low-fat diet. Genetics can also affect an individual's response to exercise, with some people seeing better results with resistance training, while others may see more significant changes with cardio.

While genetics can influence an individual's ability to lose weight, it is not the only factor that determines weight loss success. Lifestyle factors such as diet and exercise play a crucial role in achieving and maintaining a healthy weight.

Working with Your Genetics to Achieve Weight Loss

While genetics may influence an individual's weight and weight loss efforts, it is not a determining factor. Individuals can still achieve weight loss success by making lifestyle changes such as adopting a healthy diet and exercise routine.

To work with your genetics to achieve weight loss, it is essential to understand your body's specific needs. Working with a healthcare provider or nutritionist can help you identify the best diet and exercise plan for your unique needs. Additionally, tracking your progress and adjusting your plan as needed can help you achieve long-term weight loss success.

In conclusion, genetics plays a significant role in an individual's weight and weight loss efforts. However, it is not the only factor that determines weight loss success. By making lifestyle changes and working with your body's specific needs, individuals can achieve and maintain a healthy weight.

Chapter 51: The Benefits of a Balanced Diet for Weight Loss

Achieving and maintaining a healthy weight can be challenging, especially with the many fad diets and weight loss programs available in today's market. However, one of the most effective ways to reach and maintain a healthy weight is through a balanced diet. A balanced diet consists of a variety of nutrient-dense foods that provide the necessary nutrients for optimal health while also promoting weight loss.

A balanced diet typically includes a combination of fruits, vegetables, whole grains, lean protein, and healthy fats. These foods provide the body with a wide range of vitamins, minerals, and other essential nutrients that are necessary for maintaining a healthy weight. For example, fruits and vegetables are rich in fiber, which can help regulate digestion and promote feelings of fullness, reducing overall calorie intake.

Whole grains are also an essential part of a balanced diet for weight loss. Unlike refined grains, such as white bread and pasta, whole grains contain the entire grain kernel, including the bran, germ, and endosperm. This means that they are richer in fiber, vitamins, and minerals, and can help keep you feeling fuller for longer periods.

Lean protein sources, such as chicken, turkey, fish, and tofu, are also essential for weight loss. Protein has a higher thermic effect than carbohydrates or fats, meaning that the body burns more calories digesting protein than it does digesting other macronutrients. Eating a diet high in protein can also help reduce cravings and promote feelings of fullness, leading to overall reduced calorie intake.

Healthy fats, such as those found in nuts, seeds, avocados, and olive oil, are also an important part of a balanced diet for weight loss. These fats provide essential fatty acids that are necessary for optimal health and can also help promote feelings of fullness, reducing overall calorie intake.

A balanced diet can also help promote sustainable weight loss. Unlike fad diets that often involve extreme calorie restriction and elimination of entire food groups, a balanced diet provides a wide variety of foods that are enjoyable and sustainable over the long term. This means that you are more likely to stick to a balanced diet and achieve lasting weight loss results.

In addition to weight loss, a balanced diet can also provide numerous health benefits. Eating a diet rich in fruits, vegetables, whole grains, lean protein, and healthy fats can help reduce the risk of chronic diseases such as heart disease, diabetes, and certain types of cancer. It can also improve energy levels, mental clarity, and overall quality of life.

In conclusion, a balanced diet is one of the most effective ways to achieve and maintain a healthy weight. By incorporating a variety of nutrient-dense foods into your diet, you can provide your body with the necessary nutrients for optimal health while also promoting weight loss. Additionally, a balanced diet can provide numerous other health benefits, making it a sustainable and enjoyable way to achieve lasting weight loss results.

Chapter 52: The Role of Self-Compassion in Weight Loss

Losing weight can be a challenging journey, filled with ups and downs, successes, and setbacks. Many people focus solely on the physical aspects of weight loss, such as diet and exercise, while neglecting the mental and emotional factors that can play a significant role in their success. One of the most critical mental factors that can impact weight loss is self-compassion. In this chapter, we will explore the role of self-compassion in weight loss, why it matters, and how you can cultivate it to improve your chances of success.

What is Self-Compassion?

Self-compassion is the act of treating oneself with kindness, understanding, and acceptance, especially in times of difficulty or distress. It involves recognizing and acknowledging one's struggles without judgment or self-criticism. It is not the same as self-esteem, which can be tied to external factors such as success, appearance, or approval from others. Instead, self-compassion is a form of self-care and self-love that is unconditional and not dependent on outside validation.

Why Self-Compassion Matters in Weight Loss

Self-compassion is a crucial component of weight loss because it can help individuals navigate the many challenges that come with changing one's diet and exercise habits. Weight loss can be emotionally challenging, and it is common for people to experience feelings of frustration, disappointment, and even self-blame when they don't see the results they were hoping for. This negative self-talk can lead to feelings of shame, guilt, and low self-esteem, making it even harder to stay motivated and stick to healthy habits. Practicing self-compassion can help individuals break this negative cycle and approach their weight loss journey with a more positive and supportive mindset.

How Self-Compassion Supports Weight Loss

Reduces Stress: Weight loss can be stressful, and chronic stress can lead to increased levels of the hormone cortisol, which can trigger overeating and weight gain. Self-compassion can help individuals manage stress and reduce cortisol levels, making it easier to stick to healthy habits.

Increases Motivation: Self-compassion can increase motivation by fostering a sense of self-worth and self-efficacy. When individuals believe in themselves and their ability to achieve their goals, they are more likely to stick to healthy habits.

Improves Body Image: Self-compassion can improve body image by helping individuals focus on their positive qualities rather than their perceived flaws. This can lead to a more positive self-image and greater confidence, which can make it easier to stick to healthy habits.

How to Cultivate Self-Compassion for Weight Loss

Practice Mindfulness: Mindfulness involves being present in the moment and observing one's thoughts and emotions without judgment. Mindfulness can help individuals become more aware of their negative self-talk and develop a more compassionate and supportive inner voice.

Treat Yourself Like a Friend: When negative thoughts arise, ask yourself what you would say to a friend in the same situation. Treat yourself with the same kindness and understanding you would offer to someone else.

Focus on Progress, Not Perfection: Instead of focusing solely on the number on the scale, celebrate the progress you have made. Recognize that weight loss is a journey and that setbacks are a natural part of the process.

Conclusion:

Self-compassion is an essential component of weight loss that is often overlooked. By cultivating self-compassion, individuals can approach their weight loss journey with a more positive and supportive mindset, making it easier to stick to healthy habits and achieve their goals. With practice, self-compassion can become a powerful tool in your weight loss toolbox, helping you navigate the ups and downs of the journey and emerge stronger and more resilient.

Chapter 53: Conclusion and Moving Forward with Your Weight Loss Journey

Congratulations on making it this far in your weight loss journey! You've put in the hard work, dedication, and commitment to reach your goals. Now, it's time to reflect on your progress and plan for the future.

It's important to remember that losing weight is not a one-time event. It's a continuous journey that requires ongoing effort and maintenance. Therefore, it's crucial to set realistic expectations and make sustainable lifestyle changes that you can maintain in the long run.

Here are some tips for moving forward with your weight loss journey:

Celebrate your progress: Take a moment to celebrate all the hard work and progress you've made. Celebrate your milestones, big or small. This will help keep you motivated and positive about your weight loss journey.

Re-evaluate your goals: Now that you've achieved some success, it's time to re-evaluate your goals. Are they still relevant and attainable? Do you need to adjust them?

Take some time to assess your progress and adjust your goals accordingly.

Maintain healthy habits: Don't revert to your old habits. Instead, maintain the healthy habits you've developed along the way, such as eating a balanced diet, exercising regularly, and getting enough sleep. These habits will help you maintain your weight loss and improve your overall health.

Seek support: Don't be afraid to seek support from friends, family, or a professional. Weight loss can be challenging, and having someone to lean on can make all the difference.

Stay accountable: Accountability is crucial for long-term success. Keep track of your progress, and hold yourself accountable for your actions. This could mean keeping a food diary, scheduling regular workouts, or enlisting a weight loss coach.

Remember, weight loss is a journey, and it's not always going to be easy. But by celebrating your progress, re-evaluating your goals, maintaining healthy habits, seeking support, and staying accountable, you can continue to move forward with confidence and success.

www.ingramcontent.com/pod-product-compliance
Lightning Source LLC
Chambersburg PA
CBHW061603250726
48657CB00017B/1540